CURIOUS PEOPLE
COMICAL HAPPENINGS
CROWNS OF GLORY

A DENTIST'S STORY!

Barrie Lawrence

Grosvenor House
Publishing Limited

The right of Barrie Lawrence to be identified as the author of this
work has been asserted by him in accordance with Section 78
of the Copyright, Designs and Patents Act 1988

The book cover picture is copyright to Barrie Lawrence

This book is published by
Grosvenor House Publishing Ltd
28-30 High Street, Guildford, Surrey, GU1 3EL.
www.grosvenorhousepublishing.co.uk

A CIP record for this book
is available from the British Library

ISBN 978-1-78148-698-6

Cover design by Derek Blois

This book is dedicated to six amazing ladies,
who also happen to be our daughters –
each uniquely special and each greatly loved.

Sarah
Rachel
Naomi
Deborah
Fiona
Heather

We are blessed indeed!

Barrie Lawrence is also the author of -

THERE MUST BE MORE TO LIFE THAN THIS
New Wine Press (2012)

Contents

Many names have been changed in this book, but Johnny Cleveland the entertainer and comedian, is definitely Johnny Cleveland.

Foreword

Barrie Lawrence is a contradiction. He is both a dentist (now retired) and a very nice person. I rest my case!

Notwithstanding this apparent conundrum I wish to point out, from the outset, that the author of this wonderful little book is not only a thoroughly pleasant human being (indeed, some would say the archetypical 'gentleman') but also an extremely funny one. I well remember a few years ago nervously sitting in Barrie's surgery chair in Aylsham (an attractive and understated market town in Norfolk, in my opinion) about to have the first, and I hoped my last, 'bridge' inserted into my jaw and all he could focus on was the latest joke doing the rounds. It was something about Al Capone, a cat and a new pair of shoes. Truly I cannot remember the punch-line, but suffice to say it had me in stitches and my dissolving hyper-tension positively 'hissed' through his open surgery window. No doubt this was part of Barrie's professional ploy – to relax his patient before the dirty deed was done. But make no mistake, a jestful persona is very much part of who Mr. Lawrence, Dental Surgeon extraordinaire, is and those of us who are fortunate to know the man personally love him for it.

My background is a far cry from dentistry. Having studied theology at Cambridge University in the late 1980s with a view to becoming an Anglican clergyman I rapidly abandoned this idea (a long story) and, instead, embarked on a varied career including running a professional surveying business and becoming (somewhat by default) an 'expert' in things Antarctica (having walked to the South Pole in 2001 and then engaging in academic research and writing about the 'Heroic Age' of polar exploration). In addition, I have somehow found time, over the past 10 years or so, to climb a few big Nepalese and Indian Himalayan 'hills' and to be involved in a few Third World humanitarian projects along the way. I consider myself well-qualified in facing the ultimate physical and mental challenges in life - including sitting in the dreaded dentist's chair!

There are similarities here. Both Barrie and I can crack a joke or two (I would argue I am better at it!); both of us have led professional lives dealing with the challenges of business and, on occasions, some rather strange clients (as you will read in this book); and both of us share a deep faith in Christ. I was honoured to be asked by Barrie to write this preamble to his latest (and funniest) book. I have been his friend and part-time confidant for more than 15 years (goodness, how time drags!) and, therefore, feel well-placed to offer a few words of wisdom.

And what should one say of this latest Barrie Lawrence treatise?

For a start, it is a refreshingly uncomplicated, short (some might say ordinary) account of the author's life, in particular how he came to be the man with the mouth mask, bushy eyebrows, syringe and menacing hand-held high speed drill. There are some wonderful anecdotes (watch out for Barrie's tale about how he won a sherry competition; his litany of practical jokes played as a student at the London; and the Norwich patients who declared they were on 'Infidelity Benefit'). There are some most interesting insights into what is involved in becoming a qualified dentist, too (look out for the 'Phantom Heads' episode). Anyone who knows our man is fully aware of his appreciation of the fair sex and, especially, of his passion for Jesus. It shouldn't surprise us, therefore, that we discover life for 'atheist' Barrie took an interesting turn as a dental student when he met 'godly' Sheila (not quite 'when Harry met Sally', but good enough).

This wonderful little book gives us the real Barrie Lawrence. He is talented, funny, articulate, caring, generous, gracious, modest and, above all, a gifted communicator of his faith. I hate people like him, don't you? But seriously, it is so very reassuring to know that a man of such integrity is, also, just like most of us – ordinary, even a practical-joker (when the mood fits). From pretty humble beginnings and (apparently) only modest early academic promise we see a young man grow from nervous naivety into a highly-skilled professional and respected pillar of society.

Anyone who meets 'Beaming Barrie' (that's how I see him – he never fails to smile at you) will be impressed by his kindness, zest for life and, above all, his spiritual wisdom. This book encapsulates these qualities perfectly. His concern for the eternal welfare of humanity is clear for all to see. It is hardly a tome but it tells a huge story and will be enjoyed by anyone who takes the time to read it. I encourage you to find a little corner in your sitting room with a nice comfy chair to sit on, a good reading light beside you and a cup of tea in-hand (a glass of wine/sherry if Barrie has his say!) and indulge. It will be time well-spent.

Over the years I have been privileged to make some extreme journeys in this beautiful planet of ours. I was thrilled to be elected Fellow of the Royal Geographical Society in 2001 and have written extensively on the life and times of Sir Ernest Henry Shackleton (1874-1922), an Irish-born south polar explorer par excellence. At home I have a vast reference library of exploration books - mostly polar and Himalayan (by the way, does anyone know a good carpenter, the good Lord aside, as I am in desperate need of more bookshelves?). What I find fascinating in my research of all the men and women of adventure (throughout the ages) is that, for all their courage and apparent self-sufficiency, when faced with danger and/or isolation, their minds quickly turn to things 'beyond' themselves. Many feel the guiding presence of another 'invisible' being.

The young Shackleton, like Barrie in his student days, was an atheist. In 1916, at the age of 42, all that changed. When crossing the interior mountains of South Georgia, on a mission to save 22 men stranded on an uninhabited sub-Antarctic island 800 miles away, he experienced the tangible protection and reassurance of, in his words, 'a fourth presence'. Both Frank Worsley and Tom Crean, who accompanied Shackleton over this virginal frozen sub-polar terrain, had the same experience. All three only admitted this later when they came to write their memoirs. What the other two quite made of it all I do not know but for Shackleton it was a religious experience, not that he became a regular churchgoer (he was never in one place long enough).

I see clear parallels in Barrie's story. Who needs to be a polar adventurer or mountaineer to enjoy the fun and 'buzz' of living and to discover that there is something 'beyond' oneself? Being one of the best dental surgeons (retired) in Norfolk will do nicely.

Stephen Scott-Fawcett FRGS

Adventurer and Editor of the James Caird Society (London) 'Journal' and 'The Shackleton Centenary Book (2014)' ISBN 978-0-9576293-0-1 (Sutherland House Publishing).

Cromer, December 2013.

INTRODUCTION

My Arrival in the Quaint Hilltop Town of Shaftesbury, where a patient takes flight and hides in a woodyard

Neville emerged through the front door of the dental practice, heart racing and with an agitated spring in his stride. He hastened along the front path to the gate, and was soon through it and into Bleke Street. Crossing over the road and heading towards the lane curiously named Parsons Pool, he glanced over his shoulder - and froze. The dentist had opened the front door and emerged onto the path, staring across at him.

Neville increased his pace and headed along the lane, intent on getting as far from that surgery as quickly as possible. Another ten yards and he looked back again, still running. The dentist had reached the front gate, and was calling out "Come back Neville". At this the unfortunate patient felt a mighty surge of adrenaline propel him forward, and he raced along Parsons Pool.

Towards the end of the lane, where it met Bell Street, he slowed down and, assuming he was now safe, shot a glance back towards the surgery. Panic - the dentist was now in hot pursuit, white coat flowing out behind him as he raced along the lane getting ever nearer. Ahead lay the way into town, behind was the 'enemy', and to the left, the entrance to a woodyard. Without so much as a thought, Neville found himself darting into the woodyard. He dodged behind stacks of timber, and being a man of diminutive stature, soon managed to worm himself into a small space where, concealed behind some planking, he could observe the dentist now prowling up and down the yard.

* * * * * * * * * *

Nobody had told me that dental patients would ever take flight from my surgery!

I was newly qualified, and it was barely a year since I had arrived at the quaint little town of Shaftesbury in Dorset. Originally called Palladwr in Saxon times, its hilltop position gave it commanding views across the Blackmore Vale, such that one might even see Glastonbury on a clear day. And that was 40 miles away.

But I had never been told that patients might leap from the chair and run. And now this chap had really shown me a clean pair of heels.

In Roman times the name of the town had changed to Shaston, and later there had been a sizeable and hugely influential abbey, now in ruins. There was also a legend that King Arthur had burnt the cakes here, and a tea shop celebrated this and pulled in the tourists during the summer months.

I had already grown to love the town, with its curious mixture of architectural styles, uneven roof lines, narrow streets, cobbled hills, breathtaking views and more than a hint of Hardy. Indeed, just three years earlier, parts of 'Far from the Madding Crowd' had been filmed on Gold Hill in the town centre, and one half-expected to encounter Bathsheba Everdene as one strolled its streets in 1970 - though I would have settled for Julie Christie, the actress who had played the part, in those days.

So why had Neville fled? He was employed as a dish-washer at the local hotel, and had been brought to the practice by the manager there. That must have indicated a degree of apprehension in the man. The manager had brought him into the surgery itself and introduced him to me, with a "This is Neville. He feels there is something wrong with his teeth and would like you to have a look". He said he would walk back to the hotel, maybe 400 yards away, and see Neville when he returned.

Neville was a short, wiry man and sat in the chair with his mouth tightly shut. He appeared to be oblivious to me, the nurse, and his surroundings in general; in fact, he looked totally dejected.

"Good morning Neville" I said, trying to sound friendly and reassuring. But there was no reply.

"So how long have you been in Shaftesbury?" I asked, still getting no response.

"I need to know your date of birth, for the Health Service form" I said, and felt relieved when he replied "The 6th of February 1911".

If I had kept my mouth shut at this stage, it would have saved an argument, but I was not to know. "So you're 59" I said.

"No I'm not" said Neville. "I'm 53"

I considered this for a moment. "Then in that case you were born in 1917" I replied.

"No I wasn't" snapped Neville. "I was born in 1911 - on the 6th February, I was".

"Right" I said, pausing to double check my arithmetic. "1911 from 1970 is 59, so you must be 59".

Neville looked troubled by this, but then turned his head towards me and stated with defiance, "I was born in 1911, and I am 53".

There are times when one knows that logic is a waste of time, and so I quietly wrote down Neville's year of birth as 1911 and said "OK, you're 53".

I asked Neville if his teeth were at all painful, but he had his mouth tightly shut again and silently shook his head. I explained that after washing my hands I would have a look at his teeth, and tell him if I felt there was a problem.

Having washed my hands, and as I reached for the towel, Neville at last opened his mouth, uttered the words "I'm off", and leaping from the chair, careered out of the surgery.

I just stared at the empty chair and the open door. I still felt such a novice, and turned to the nurse and asked "What do I do now?" Sarah had been at the practice for a couple of years or so, and I relied so much on her knowledge of 'what to do next', but she just shrugged her shoulders and looked blank.

As we stood there trying to weigh up the situation, Neville shot back into the surgery, grabbed his overcoat from the back of the door, and with the explanation "want m' coat", flew out of the surgery for a second time. I went to the window, and saw him cross the road and break into an energetic stroll as he entered the road opposite, called Parsons Pool.

A quick glance at my list of patients for the day confirmed that I was still significantly underbooked, and had no more patients for nearly an hour. I decided that I had nothing to lose in pursuing Neville, and so with a view to persuading him to let me put his teeth right, and still wearing my white coat, I emerged from the front door of the practice and called out after him. Neville took one look over his shoulder, and immediately broke into a run. I hardly paused for thought as I dashed over the road, and with my white coat streaming out behind me, gave chase to the unfortunate patient.

Neville glanced over his shoulder again, gasped, and tore along Parsons Pool with me hot on his heels. It was not a long road, and at the end, on the left hand side, was the entrance to the woodyard. Here Neville skidded to a halt, and without looking back, darted through the gateway. By the time I reached the entrance, there was no sign of the man, and so I paced slowly up and down, calling out "Neville, where are you?", and looking round the corners created by the numerous stacks of timber.

Two workmen came out of an office and asked if they could help, staring at my white coat. "I've lost a patient" I explained. "He's hiding in your woodyard somewhere".

They looked completely non-plussed and told me to feel free to search for the man, and then retreated into the workshop, whispering to each other.

And there I will leave the story for now. But Neville did find himself back in the surgery, and well within the hour at that. He also continued to return for a lengthy course of treatment, only to experience a dental disaster a very short time later. And the background was almost unbelievable, but that I will come to as well.

I have precious memories of those early days in Shaftesbury - of the excitement of starting out as a dentist in that enchanting country town, of the people, rich in character, who were to cross my path and pass through my surgery, and of incidents that still cause me to smile as I reflect upon them. And there are memories of the early days of marriage to my University sweetheart, our first rented home that was virtually bare due to a strike at the furniture factory, and the birth of our first two beautiful daughters.

But why does anybody decide to be a dentist, and what train of events led to me starting work in Shaftesbury, and chasing a patient into a woodyard?

Read on!

CHAPTER 1

Leeches in the bedroom, a frog in the toilet, and a booklet that determined my future

I left the careers exhibition clutching a booklet that had a tasteful olive green cover. It was entitled 'Dentistry - A Career and a Future', by Mr. Neil Livingstone-Ward. I could never have guessed that five years later I would be taught dentistry by Mr. Neil Livingstone-Ward.

My paternal grandparents lived in Peterborough, and their house backed onto the showground. It was still quite a journey round to the showground entrance, but Grandpa had adjusted the wooden fencing such that, with sliding two bolts, some of the slats swung open to give us access (and with no entrance fee) to the showground. I recalled that this had been our entrance many years before when we had gone to the circus, and the clowns had frightened me, and made me cry! And today we had passed through the fence yet again, and Grandpa had guided me around the exhibition, browsing the various stalls and presentations, until we came to the 'Dentistry' display.

But it wasn't the tasteful olive green colour of the cover, nor the title, nor yet the rather posh name of the author - it was the picture! The title was at the top, and the author's name at the bottom, and in the centre of the cover was a photograph. And that was the deciding factor - a dentist in the cleanest white coat you can imagine, working in a state-of-the-art surgery. The patient was gazing up, admiringly, over her right shoulder, and there in the corner of the surgery, was the cutest little dolly-bird of a nurse that I had ever seen. I took one look at the photograph and decided, "I'm going to be a dentist!"

* * * * * * * * * *

And yet this was the culmination of years of preparation, during which the future direction of my life had, at least in general terms, been determined.

"I don't mind you going out into the countryside," said my mother, "But do you have to bring so much of it back into our home?"

She called my bedroom my 'menagerie' or 'little zoo', and I never denied that there were quite a lot of animals living there. I had caught the frog by a stream, and it now had a reasonably happy existence in a relatively large jar by my bed. And yet, although there was water in the jar, it would choose a time when I was absent from the bedroom, and jump out and make for the toilet, where it would sit absolutely motionless on the loo seat. The first time this happened it took me a while to find it, as it was so very still and my eye passed over the creature without noticing it. But after that first time, I knew where to look. And there was also my mother's voice, calling out to my sister, "Julia. Use the downstairs toilet this morning."

There was a mill pond a few miles out of town, and that supplied me with pond skaters, water boatmen, water snails, and a host of other aquatic specimens. My butterfly net also yielded three different species of leech from the same pond, but I found to my dismay that they 'ate' the water snails in my aquarium. So each species of leech was kept in a separate water-filled jam jar, and fed on garden snails.

Stick insects were present in many a schoolboy's bedroom in those days (so I told my mother), but the wild field mice were almost unique to my room. I had caught them myself, and was quite proud of the method I and my friend John had devised for catching them. We would cycle to harvested fields outside the nearby village of Felmingham, and identify the new stacks with bales of straw lying on the ground around the stack itself. I preferred to be the 'catcher', and would position myself by a bale. On the word 'Go', John would pick up the bale as best he could, and I would fall onto the exposed ground, directing myself towards any 'squeak', and hopefully landing on a mouse. Indeed, if I felt a wriggling under my tummy, I knew I had been successful. With my gloves firmly in place, I would slide my hands under my stomach and grab anything that wriggled and place it in my coat pocket, to be transferred to the dry aquarium when I reached home again. And so the collection built up, and at the same time John and I became famous amongst our peers as 'mousers'.

"Oh No! He's got a snake," said my sister, as the slow worm slithered out of my blazer pocket. I had paid a shilling for it from another boy at school, and it became resident in my room for a few months. The slow worm is a lizard without legs, but I could forgive the family for thinking it was a snake.

One other aspect of my life at this time touches on a matter of historical interest. It was the very early 1960s and farmers were noticing that when their crops first appeared as green shoots, they did not remain so for long. They were being eaten, and at a rate never known before. Furthermore, when the farmers walked round their fields to investigate, and particularly those fields adjoining rivers and streams, they were liable to fall through the surface of the ground into large subterranean burrows. The culprits were found to be coypus, large rodents that had escaped from farms where they were being bred for their fur. At this time I was studying for my 'A' level GCEs and needed to dissect rats, which were supplied to the school by the education authority. However, there was a shortage at that time, and so I took it upon myself to supply the school with rats, and I and my friend John obtained some gin traps which we took to the water meadows of Tuttington, a small rural village a few miles from where we lived. There we would easily distinguish in the grass the runs through which the coypus would traverse the meadows, and set three or four of the traps. We would then wander along the river bank, often stopping to watch the coypus surfacing in the water and playing around on the opposite bank. A little after sunset we would return to our traps, and generally find we had caught at least two or three of the creatures. They were rife at that time, and were a considerable size, measuring around 1 metre (39 inches) from their muzzle to the tip of their tail. We would take strong cord with us, and having killed the creatures, would tie their front legs together and then suspend them by their legs from the handlebars of our bicycles. Whilst doing this, I would try and hold the saddle of the bike down, as the weight of just one coypu would cause the back of the bike to rear in the air as the handle bars crashed down. Sometimes I would set off for home, cycling along the narrow Norfolk roads, with two huge 'rats' swinging from the handlebars, now and then being caught in the headlights of an oncoming car, and wondering what on earth the driver would think of the curly headed boy pedalling along with enormous rodents swinging from the front of his bike. Incidentally, the coypu is not a rat, though generally referred to in Norfolk at that time as 'great old rats' (and in the local dialect), but a close relative of the capybara, the largest living rodent and, like the coypu, a native of South America. Also, they were quite harmless unless cornered, being herbivorous, though many a Norfolk soul had the life frightened out of them by a show of long yellow incisor teeth and a fearsome snarling sound.

* * * * * * * * * *

So the careers exhibition was really the final determining factor in my choice of career, but there was one other aspect that seemed significant at the time. My mother kept asking me what I was going to do with my life, and I replied that I wanted to do something with natural history. David Attenborough was starting to become prominent on the television, searching Borneo for a dragon in those days, I believe, and I felt inspired. My mother explained to me that this was not really a practical option for 'people like us', and so I tried to think of other careers that involved biology and zoology to some extent.

My father was a bank clerk, and it was assumed that I would do something similar. In fact, when most of my contemporaries left school at the age of sixteen, approximately half of my school year went to work at the Norwich Union, a large insurance company of national significance based in our local city of Norwich. I did not think 'money' and I did not think 'professions', though my father tried to put me right on these two scores. We were not too comfortable financially at times, with my father having had considerable periods of time off work with nervous breakdowns. Most of the time we were able to have a car, and my father would drive us down to the coast in the summer, but there were times when we were not so well off and the family would walk or cycle places, though those times were relatively few. So my father realized the significance of money, from working in a bank and seeing how much other people had, and also from not having enough himself at times, which explained why there were those occasions when he would arrive home at the end of the day, and after having put his black bicycle away in the shed, sit down and exclaim "No wonder we haven't got any money. The doctors and dentists have it all."

I do not think those words really bore fruit with me, but having said that, I can still recall them half a century later. And so with perhaps a little steering from my parents, I decided that I should be a biology teacher, a vet, a doctor, or a dentist.

"Not a teacher," said my mother, who had a rather low opinion of that profession. So I was not to be a teacher.

I considered being a vet (like my friend John had decided – him of 'mousing fame'), but recalled that when I was young, my mother had always told me to be very careful of dogs, and if at all possible, to avoid them altogether. Why? "Because they bite you," was always her reply. And when I considered vets, I saw in my mind dogs and cats, and especially dogs. And I knew that they could bite you. So I was not to be a vet.

The idea of being a doctor was not without its attractions, as my parents seemed to revere that profession and felt they were on a somewhat higher plane than the rest of humanity. Maybe I could attain to such a lofty position in society, though I had no idea of the training or qualifications required. But one thing I did know was that when I was very young and living in Hertfordshire, Dr. MacDonald-Smith had turned out in the middle of the night (well, I was about six years of age and had gone to bed) to examine my spots and announce that I had chicken pox. I had no intention of following a career that involved getting up in the middle of the night, and so I was not to be a doctor.

And that left 'dentist'.

Shortly after this I went to the careers exhibition at Peterborough, which finalized the decision.

And at the age of around fifteen, this was exactly what I needed – to know what I wanted in life, because it gave me direction and motivation. Firstly, instead of generally thinking that I would like to do biology, I now knew that I needed passes in five 'O' level GCEs including English and Maths, and that I would then need to pass Zoology, or Biology, together with Physics and Chemistry at 'A' level, in order to embark on my training at dental school. So my studying became more focussed.

Secondly, having made a career choice, I now knew not only what subjects I needed to study, but also that I needed to gain passes at a certain level in them. This was motivation indeed, and there was less mousing, less time spent dipping nets into ponds, and less time spent indulging in what I and my friends had come to call 'bird watching', which had nothing whatsoever to do with ornithology and everything to do with sitting in a cafe in town and gawping at the girls walking past. Instead, a card table was erected in my bedroom, and I would sit and study books and old examination papers until midnight for at least five evenings a week.

Which is all so different from the world of today, where I would ask young people coming into my surgery what career they were aiming for, only to be given a blank stare, or at most a grunt of "I don't know." But times have changed, and maybe these teenagers are much more flexible in adapting to a far more fluid employment situation.

And to be fair, just once in a while a teenaged patient would look me in the eye and tell me, "I want to be a dentist." I would always suggest that they joined me at the practice for a few days, and the wannabe dentist would arrive and excitedly don a white coat that was usually far too big for them, and come into the surgery where they could observe and generally assist in the role of trainee nurse. One young man had an almost perpetual grin as he gazed over my shoulder into a variety of mouths day by day, and positively enthused over blood. He was quite short, and though the white coat in which he was cloaked reached down to his ankles and caused him to resemble a Dalek, was known affectionately by the staff as 'Dr. Who.'

But I had not yet been accepted by a dental school, and because I had always been so mediocre academically, it was debatable as to whether I would, in fact, make it.

CHAPTER 2

Latin, The Dam Busters Man, and a Cube of Hard Yellow Wax!

"I wish I was a dentist," said the young man in dirty jeans as he climbed into my chair, and then made some allusion to the white Lotus Esprit parked by the front of the practice.

Back in the early 60s, sitting at my card table surrounded by text books on zoology, chemistry and physics, and gazing out of the bedroom window into the vegetable patch in the back garden of our home in North Walsham, I would never have dreamed that twenty years later I would really be a dentist, and as for a Lotus.........

I had always struggled academically, and if it had not been for intensive coaching by my mother (for which I will always be grateful), I would not have passed my Eleven Plus examination. The Eleven Plus examination determined whether one's secondary education would be primarily academic, or lean more towards technical skills. Despite the intensive coaching, I was deemed to be a borderline case, and had to retake the examination. At the second attempt I passed and therefore went to a grammar school, where I continued to struggle with English, mathematics, history, geography and sciences. I preferred mousing!

However, the day would come when my academic mediocrity would prove to be an advantage, though this would not be until the end of my fifth year at grammar school. For four of those five years I had been in the 'A' stream, coming bottom, after coming towards the top in the 'B' stream in my first year. At the end of that fifth year we all took our 'O' (Ordinary) level GCE examinations, and a few weeks later I gathered with most of the rest of my year to watch the results pinned up on the school notice board. I needed five passes including English and maths in order to remain on course for dental school, and with great relief found that I had not only met the requirements, but had, in fact, passed all seven subjects taken. There were no grade 1s or Distinctions in subjects such as most of my peers had achieved, but I simply had seven mediocre passes.

It was nearly a year later, as we approached the summer prize day that I felt someone at the school had made a big mistake. I received a letter asking me to name which book, or books, up to a certain value I would like to receive as my prize for coming first in Five Science the previous year. I went and saw the school secretary to explain there had been a mistake, only to listen in sheer amazement as she explained that I was the only boy in the class to pass in *all* seven 'O' level subjects. Others had a clutch of distinctions, but only I had seven passes. And so for the first and only time in my seven years at that school, I marched across the stage (the school had a military history and style) and shook hands with Sir Barnes Wallis, the inventor of the bouncing bomb of Dam Busters fame, not to mention the Wellington bomber, and collected a couple of books on zoology. And then it was back to school lessons, dissecting coypus, and sitting at that card table evening after evening.

And so I started thinking seriously about training to be a dentist, and though there were dental schools in most of the major cities in the UK, I felt that London was the place for a lad from rural Norfolk to see what life was all about. This was something of a disappointment for my mother, who had wanted me to study at either Oxford or Cambridge and who had nailed her colours to the mast as I approached the start of the fourth year at school.

Upon entering the fourth form, certain decisions had to be made with regard to the emphasis of one's education, and we were given the option of doing just one of the following four subjects – Latin, art, woodwork or music. I felt that art would be fun, and said that would be my decision. "No," said my grandmother, and explained that we had many musicians in the family, and I should do music.

"You're doing Latin," said my mother, and explained that a pass in Latin was a requirement for entering Oxford and Cambridge Universities, and she rather hoped that I might go to one of them. Not that any one else in our family had ever gone to *any* University! So I studied Latin, only to find a few years later that firstly, the requirement to pass Latin was dropped by both Universities, and secondly, there were no dental schools in either Oxford or Cambridge.

I applied to each of the dental schools attached to major teaching hospitals in London, and duly went for interview at each. Interviews were usually conducted by the dean or subdean, and one of the questions asked was "Why do you want to be a dentist." The fact that this question was usually asked was made clear in most of the booklets and pamphlets one could obtain to prepare oneself for the interviews, together with the fact that the interviewers were looking for students who 'liked doing things with their hands.' This almost certainly accounted for the results of a later survey that showed that in answer to that question, over 50% of interviewees replied, "Because I like doing things with my hands."

"Just what do you like doing with your hands?" I was asked at each of the five interviews, and proceeded to talk about my model-making (mainly aircraft) and the hours I spent with my fretsaw making, well, tooth brush holders seemed worth a mention. I decided to keep quiet about the fact that I caught mice with my hands. At one interview we were all given a solid cube of very hard yellow wax, along with a knife, and told to carve it into a pyramid. It looked like the hardest of cheese, and seemed to have the hardness of glass. My little knife kept skidding down the sides and if the winner had been the one with the most shavings..... but that was not the case, and my very unkempt offering may well have contributed to me coming away with a provisional place, and not a definite one.

Most of the dental schools put me on their provisional list, which meant that if enough of those students given a firm place failed, I would be given a place if I passed my 'A' levels. However, the London Hospital in Whitechapel gave me a firm place, so long as I passed my three 'A' (Advanced) levels in zoology, chemistry and physics.

And so it was back to the card table in the bedroom till midnight almost every night, and back to the dissection room in the biology laboratory at school until the two years of study were over and it was time to take the 'A' level examinations. The results were understandably a while coming through, and so I cycled off each day to nearby farms where I picked broad beans, blackcurrants, strawberries and anything else in season in order to have a little money to take to London with me, should I have the necessary 'A' level passes. In fact, the largest farm in the area thought I might be useful in other ways, and offered me employment for the rest of the summer, which I spent pruning raspberry canes, weighing other peoples' broad beans, blackcurrants and strawberries, as well as cleaning out broiler houses. Broiler houses were long low buildings in which thousands of chickens jostled together in deep straw until they were slaughtered for meat. After that a pair of us would enter the building, with masks to protect us from the intense smell of ammonia, and brush the filthy straw, heavy with excrement and dead rotting chickens, out of the house. After cycling the seven miles home in the evening I would get in the bath, submerge for a minute or so, and upon surfacing, see how many bugs and similar were floating on the water.

The fateful day arrived when 'A' level students crowded round the notice board back at school, and I gave a great sigh of relief to find that my mediocrity had again carried me through, for though my grades would never get me into a dental school today, I had managed a pass in each which secured me a place back in 1963. I was soon on the telephone informing the London Hospital that I had my necessary passes, and my parents were delighted to think that their son might one day be a dentist.

CHAPTER 3

The Elephant Man, the Elephant's Teeth, the Kray Brothers, and a Fifty-Six Mile Stroll

For a Norfolk lad, setting out for London was quite an adventure, especially in those days when Norfolk seemed so insular. There are many parts of the UK that people pass through when travelling from A to B, but nobody passes through Norfolk. My home county is on a bulge on the eastern side of England, and to the north and east is the North Sea. There were no motorways serving the area then, or now, and so we tended to be rather isolated. I lived in a small town called North Walsham, and people wanting to go to department stores would travel the 10 miles or so to the city of Norwich, which though small for a city, seemed like a metropolis because it was our *only* city. I recall two men in their twenties deciding to have an exciting day out and to travel down to London, a little over a hundred miles away, and of which most people had only heard stories. For some reason they were unable to travel at the same time on the same train, and so agreed that they would meet 'in London outside the post office'. Upon arrival, each found a post office, but unlike North Walsham, there was more than one post office. In fact there were scores, probably hundreds, which was way beyond the comprehension of many a Norfolk man at that time. They never met each other in London that day!

There was a friendly soul called Charlie who used to do some gardening for my parents on occasions. He was a simple man, of great girth and with a perpetual rosy-cheeked smile. Charlie fell in love with Martha, who cleaned some of the classrooms at our school, and they were well-suited to each other, with matching smiles, intellects and figures. Most local couples went to the coast, around 5 miles away, and spent their honeymoons in a caravan, but Charlie decided that he was going to honeymoon in style, and booked a place in Kings Lynn, around 50 miles away. Upon his return, he was fêted as North Walsham's answer to Marco Polo, as he sat in the coffee bar and related stories of his time in Kings Lynn – of the way the people spoke with their strange accent, of the food they ate, and of their curious customs. And the locals hung on his every word.

* * * * * * * * * *

I arrived in London in September 1963, with two huge suitcases and a map of the London Underground. My destination was Commonwealth Hall, a recently-opened University Hall of Residence, for men only (the girls hall of residence was next door), situated in Cartwright Gardens in central London. I found my way there on the Underground, known as the 'Tube', announced my arrival at reception and was given forms to fill in. My room was number G4 on the ground floor (there were 8 floors in all), and I had a bed, desk, desk chair and easy chair. It smelt new. This hall became my home for the next 18 months or so, and my life here broadened my education more than I could ever have imagined. There were students from all parts of the UK and of the world, and of all ethnicities, studying every subject imaginable (though there seem to be far more today). Sitting down to dinner one evening during my first week there, and having introduced myself to the chap sitting opposite me, and learnt that his name was Simon, I asked him where he was from. He asked me if I was familiar with England, and if so, did I know where Norfolk was. Simon lived around 10 miles from me. "Small world," we said, but many of the other people I became friendly with were from places as distant as the USA and the Punjab.

* * * * * * * * * *

But of even more interest to me at this point, was the hospital where I was to study, learn, and train to be a dentist for the next five years. The London Hospital, known to all those who worked and studied there simply as 'the London', was situated in the east end of London in the district of Whitechapel. The name Whitechapel is well known to a large proportion of the British population; to board game aficionados, it is the cheapest property on the monopoly board, whilst to readers of ghoulish non-fiction crime stories it is the area in which Jack the Ripper (possibly a surgeon at 'the London') tore the life out of a number of ladies of ill repute in the late 19th century; and then again to students of other ghoulish non-fiction literature, it was the area where John Merrick, real name Joseph Merrick, the Elephant Man lived. Joseph Merrick had such facial deformities that he was paraded as a human curiosity in the latter half of the 19th century, and his skull was an exhibit in our dental museum at the hospital.

But in the 1960s when the curly-haired young man from Norfolk arrived as a student in the area, these colourful characters from Whitechapel's history were well gone. However, the vacuum they left had been filled by two brothers, Ronnie and Reggie Kray. They were boxers, turned gangsters, and everybody seemed to know them personally. Reggie was well spoken of by most people, whereas Ronnie was generally known as a psychopath ("Not normal, pulling out a gun and blowing holes in the ceiling, it's not"), though there were many who were suspicious of *both* of them ("Not normal for boys to strangle cats for fun, it's not"). I never met either of them, though one evening, just after 8 p.m. on 9th March 1966, I walked along Whitechapel Road and passed a public house called the Blind Beggar. Twenty minutes later a car drew up at the kerb, a man got out and stepped into the public house. 'Bang!' - a single bullet just above the right eye from a Luger pistol killed George Cornell, a member of a rival gang to the Krays called the Richardsons. Ronnie Kray calmly strolled back to the car and drove off, but nobody saw a thing. Of course they didn't! And local people kept telling me about 'poor old George', because it was a close-knit community and everybody knew him.

With briefcase in hand, I made the twenty minute journey on the London Underground to the station of Whitechapel, where I disembarked and ascended a number of steps to emerge on the Whitechapel Road, opposite the hospital where I was to study, examine, inject, fill, extract, and romance my future wife for the next five years. I followed the directions sent to me a week or so earlier and found myself in a large hallway, where other young men, and three or four ladies, were clearly as new to the place as I was. There were just twenty of us, and we were called 'Blue Year'. We filled in forms, were photographed, underwent a medical check, and were given a tour of the college.

The hospital had a fine history, being founded in 1740 and having the first medical college in England and Wales in 1785. Household names such as Edith Cavell and Dr. Barnardo had worked there, and many other doctors and surgeons who were eminent in their day, and whose names continue to be used to describe sicknesses and diseases. Opposite the hospital was the Whitechapel street market, where the somewhat scruffy stallholders were said to return home at the end of the day in their Rolls Royces, discretely parked in side streets. But to most Whitechapel residents, the London was 'our hospital', and staff and students were treated with great warmth and respect.

Blue Year was a diverse group, mainly from the UK but with the West Indies and South America represented, comprising sixteen men and four ladies. For my part, I came to deeply appreciate the different personalities within Blue Year – the extroverts who laughed loudly and were the life of every party, and those of us who were from the backwoods of the UK and who shyly listened in. We were the final year of twenty, and from the following year there were around fifty students in a year, accommodated in a new Dental Institute where we all learned dentistry in state of the art dental units. But we were a small group, and as such each of us had the opportunity to get to know everybody else.

David Lucas was the youngest person ever to gain entry to a UK dental school and destined for a distinguished career. He was also on a full government grant, and his proclamation of this did not sit comfortably with those whose parents were having to support them, and led to immediate friction. Around half our number had been educated at public schools, and Barry Patten's cut-glass accent, and Martin Meadow's smooth manner set them apart in a way of which they themselves were largely unaware, and one of the ladies was said to be a descendant of *the* Asquith. Mike Grant looked too young to have left school, and yet was the only person engaged to be married. Pete Giordano enjoyed the reputation of being an ace womaniser (so he kept telling us) whereas Bari Pitt kept himself so separate that no one really got to know him at all. Nandi Maharana was the perfect gentleman, and though he was to succeed *par excellence* as a dentist, could probably have made as good a living by placing money on horses. Ron Bateman had been a dental technician, and was retraining as he had decided he wanted more clinical involvement. He was a decade ahead of the rest of us, and when we celebrated our 21st birthdays, Ron celebrated his 31st. I enjoyed the company of each and every one of them, and though I rarely meet them today, fifty years on there is still something of a 'family feel' about those who I spent five of my formative years with.

Our tour of the hospital and college was extensive - and much of it largely forgotten today. Prior to the tour we assembled in a large hallway, and after waiting some time, a few of us sat on the lower end of a wide staircase. I found myself beside John Large, and we were soon engaged in conversation, with me chatting away about the wilds of rural Norfolk and John telling me of how he had lived all his life in north London. He told me he was Jewish, and I had to confess that I had never met any Jewish person before. "There's quite a few of us in this group", he told me. "Amazing", I responded, having only read about such people in the Bible up to that point. In fact the hospital had been largely founded and funded by Jewish people and with Jewish finance, and Whitechapel in the 1960s was still a Jewish area. I don't think I met one of their number who did not have a warm and engaging personality (though I never met the Kray brothers), and I was to benefit from the generosity of one Jewish family in particular.

I remember well being shown the dissection room. "What do we dissect?" asked he of previous 'mousing' fame, and was told by the man with an Oxford accent, "The human body, of course". And there in the dissection room were around 20 tables, each with a sheet covering an object of, well, irregular shape, though almost recognisably human. And on lifting the corner of a sheet, we could discern the somewhat leathery cadaver that had once been a living person. We were told that we would be dissecting the head, neck, thorax and abdomen, but that the medical students would be removing the arms and legs for their own studies. No one asked where the cadavers came from, though there were rumours that some were vagrants who died in the wards, or people who had nobly donated their bodies for this purpose.

At the end of the room a skeleton hung from a hook on a wrought iron stand. The skeleton was that of Frederick Nicholas Charrington, a member of the well-known brewing family who had become an evangelical Christian and philanthropist. He died in the London Hospital in 1936 and donated his body for medical research. The medical and dental students who had benefitted from this 'donation' were innumerable.

At the end of the tour we were addressed by a senior member of the dental school. We were now members of the London, and any previous loyalty to school should be laid down in favour of the hospital. We were training to be members of a profession, and should dress, act, speak and present ourselves accordingly. To the men – you shave in the morning and not in the evening; *navvies* shave in the evening.

Looking back to that day and the period of time it represented, I feel the change in culture with regard to those working in the professions has been a retrograde step. Doctors, dentists, accountants, solicitors, and others largely dress casually, with jeans, rugby shirts, trainers and such like. Not all, but many. There was a time when a man with the toothache would go to the barber, who dressed like a barber, and carried out the work of a dentist. Crudely. But from around 1921, the year of the Dentists Act, that changed, and dentistry became a profession, and those practicing it dressed, acted, spoke and presented themselves as such. Today, many dentists dress, act, speak and present themselves as barbers. (But I'm sure the treatment they dispense is excellent, if cost is an indication!) In fact, all but one of our year wore a jacket and tie daily – except Mr. Casual, who shall remain nameless, and who always wore a black roll top under his corduroy jacket.

And then it was off to the canteen, where students and staff could purchase lunch at an extremely competitive price. Alongside the roasts and pies, they sold cigarettes. But that was the 1960s, and many of us smoked in those days, even in the canteen - smokers sitting amongst non-smokers who were eating.

Drugs? I never heard of any students using drugs in those days, though the tramps on the streets of Whitechapel were often addicted to methylated spirits. They would mix it with water, shaking it up in a bottle, and then sit in graveyards consuming it together. Their brains were affected by this abuse, and I often passed such an addict completely out of his mind and shouting into the air.

The dental course would involve live patients, on whom we would inject gums, fill and extract teeth, make dentures and so much more. However, before the hospital would let us loose in that manner, we had to complete a preclinical year.

Preclinical - nothing involving clinics, or patients, or real treatment. It sounded rather boring, and to some extent it was. And yet there was the novelty of that year - life in the big city, with new friends and a new environment. We learnt about anatomy - where is the heart and what is its size, where are the lungs and what is their size, where is the pancreas and what is its size, and so on and so forth. We learnt about physiology - what is the heart and what does it do, what is a lung and what does it do, what is the pancreas and what does it do, and so on and so forth.

And of course, we learnt about dental anatomy - how many teeth does an anteater have, and what are they like? (It doesn't have any). How many teeth does a crocodile have, and what are they like? (Variable, recurved). How many teeth does an elephant have, and what are they like? (I've forgotten, but I think they're big). And eventually we were taught about human teeth (thirty two - incisors, canines, premolars and molars) and the structure of teeth themselves (enamel, dentine, cementum, and pulp). We were not taught, but guessed, that the pulp was the bit that patients called 'the nerve' and usually said "Please don't 'it it!"

* * * * * * * * * *

Hospital life involved a great deal of study, with lectures and dissection during the days, and a certain amount of 'homework' to be completed in the evenings. However, I was also introduced to a social life that was completely outside my previous experience.

My life back in Norfolk had been largely home-centred. My parents rarely had alcohol - it was too expensive. My father had smoked cigarettes as a younger man, but had given the habit up. My social life at home had consisted of golf occasionally (with my father), rifle shooting sometimes (with my father), and the local youth club (where I would sometimes have, and meet up with, a girlfriend). Otherwise I was studying.

But now all that was changing. Together with some of my friends at home, I had indulged in the occasional smoke outside the youth club. Now I was free to smoke at will, and found that many of my fellow dental students did so - I joined them, and soon had a favourite brand. At home I had consumed the occasional half pint of brown ale with friends from the youth club, but at the dental school I found that to visit the Sammie (The Good Samaritan public house situated immediately behind the hospital and frequented almost exclusively by hospital staff and students) at the end of the day was considered by many of my fellow students to be quite 'normal'. However, my consumption of both tobacco and cigarettes was limited by the rather modest government grant I was receiving - but life was so very different now!

There were parties, usually given by those students who were renting flats, and generally at weekends. I always took a bottle, but seemed to drink so much more. Where did it all come from? And we would dance and dance until alcohol and exertion rendered us fit only for bed. And so late. The House of the Rising Sun by the Animals was a favourite number on the record player, and was played incessantly at some of those parties, followed at a later hour by Francoise Hardy when the smoochy ones were appropriate.

Dental Dinners were the first formal dinners I had attended, and I soon learnt what a dinner jacket was and where to hire one. They were also the wildest I would ever attend. Staff and students would be there, and indeed were expected to be. Those of exalted position, such as the dean and subdean, not to mention professors and consultants from every department, with their senior registrars in train, would attend both at the cocktail reception that preceded the dinner proper, and then at the table. There was an air of dignity as the exalted ones stood to give speeches - forgotten today, and largely forgotten a few minutes after they were delivered.

But there was an air of mischievous excitement at the first of those dinners, concerning, so it seemed, the fact that a senior registrar in the dental clinic, who always enthused over being known as 'one of the boys', had thrown out a general challenge to be 'debagged'. This was a mystery to me, but was clearly expected to be the very climax of the evening's proceedings. After the speeches, there was a general drift from the table towards the bar, when there was a great shout of "Get him!" Almost immediately there appeared to be a massive rugby scrum, with shouting, laughing, screaming and fumbling as around twenty or more of the dignified ones dived onto those already involved.

The dean and subdean looked at each other and said "NOT this year", and proceeded to stride into the melee and grab the back of the collar of whoever was nearest, and as they pulled them free from the 'scrum', uttered with surprise and disgust "Professor Henderson-Jones!" and "Dr. Masterson-Smith!" and "Professor Barrington-McKay" and so on until only one man remained - the now trouserless senior registrar who had thrown down the challenge, who with raucous laugh ran with a drunken lurch out of the restaurant door, wearing only his shirt and underpants. As I said earlier, these dinners were the first *formal* dinners that I had attended.

* * * * * * * * * *

I had heard about 'The Brighton Walk' shortly after arriving at the London, maybe through publicity at one of the Fresher's Evenings where we were encouraged to walk around the different stalls and displays advertising the various societies, associations and other activities that one could get involved in at the college. Apparently many years previously some medical students who were newly qualified decided to celebrate the occasion by walking from London to Brighton. Their route was the main road leading down to the south coast, the A23, and the distance was around 56 miles, so we were told (though I have read more recently that it is now 54 miles, probably due to the road having been greatly modified and taking a more direct route in places today). The students involved in that first ever Brighton Walk had decided that in order to enhance the celebratory nature of the walk, they would stop at every public house on the way. By the time I entered the London, the sponsors of the walk, Guinness (makers of a stout ale of that name) and Ovaltine (makers of a bedtime drink) had dropped any reference to the original nature of the walk, but I and some of my colleagues had not!

Medical and dental students from almost every one of the large number of hospitals in London gathered at Tower Bridge at 6 p.m. on a Friday evening, and numbered well in excess of 2,000. Those of us at the centre or rear did not hear the 'Go', but were soon flowing with the crowd, streaming away from the bridge and heading south. I and my small group of friends very soon reached our first public house, and called in for a quick half pint of beer. And before long we had reached the second, and then the next....... It was not too long before I realised I had lost touch with my companions, and only later found out that they had soon given up and caught an Underground train home.

It soon became obvious to me that even in the company of friends, stopping at every public house from London to Brighton was not a very practical idea, and I decided to just walk. I would walk, walk, walk, and eventually I would arrive at Preston Park in Brighton. But another problem soon presented itself – Barrie's bladder. The lad from the backwoods of Norfolk could not have imagined the distance involved in simply walking out of London, and the number of pubs was beyond my comprehension. I was uncomfortable, and there seemed to be a dearth of public conveniences beside the A23 as I plodded on through the southern suburbs of London. But there were trees, and I was becoming desperate. And so I used a tree, making sure I was positioned away from any approaching vehicle..... until another vehicle approached from the opposite direction. It had been dark for some time, and it was rather like being centre stage with the spotlights on me.

Halfway to Brighton I arrived at Gatwick, where one of the sponsors had set up a soup kitchen. I was tired and weary after 28 miles of trudge, and soup seemed like more than a good idea. I thankfully took a mug of chicken soup, and sat down on the grass verge and slowly sipped through it. Soup – a good idea. Sitting down for twenty minutes – a bad idea. It took an age to get back on my feet, and then there was the exertion of sheer willpower in order to get moving again. I was so very stiff, and it was painful, but the longer I kept moving, the easier it became.

Seventeen hours and forty-five minutes after leaving Tower Bridge, I arrived in Brighton. I was exhausted, and declined the fried breakfast that was still being offered to that tiny minority who were coming in, but had a long cool drink and headed for one of the coaches that was waiting to take us back to London. I was almost immediately asleep, and after arriving back in the big city, could hardly get myself off the coach, and with great difficulty hobbled slowly to the nearest Underground station. Back at Commonwealth Hall I spent much of the weekend in bed.

I was glad to have completed the walk, and there was a reward. Firstly, there was a green tie emblazoned with toucans, the logo of Guinness, and, secondly, there was a luncheon at the Park Royal brewery where Guinness and Harp Lager was produced. It was a great meal, and every time my lager glass became empty, it was filled again immediately without enquiry. I shall never know how many glasses of Harp Lager I consumed that lunch time, or how I got to the underground station in order to get home. But it was a memorable journey, and the one and only time a train has been stopped by the guard in order to eject the lad from Norfolk.

I took part in the walk again the following two years, though I had learnt my lesson well the previous year. Firstly, I did not stop at any public houses on the way, and secondly I decided that the best way to tackle it was to walk ten miles, run ten miles, walk ten miles and so on. And I was not to stop, at all. By the third time, I had changed very much as a person – but that too we will come to shortly. Suffice it to say that I completed the 'walk' in a little over fourteen hours on each of the two subsequent occasions, and enjoyed a wonderful luncheon out at Park Royal. I was also able to sport a maroon tie (second year), and then a grey tie (third year), as a sign of my achievement.

Tragically on that third year, a medical student was in collision with a car and died as a result. It was suggested that he had consumed quite a large number of pain killers, but the sponsors felt that, whatever the reason, the walk should be discontinued. This was in the mid-1960s when the roads were far less busy than today, but after some years a cross-country walk was launched in place of the previous Brighton Walk. But that was after my time.

* * * * * * * * * *

But there was one event that first term at the London which was to affect the direction of my future life in a major way, and that was the Fresher's Hop. A hop? That was the name given to a dance evening at the hospital, and at the beginning of each academic year, either in late September or early October, there would be such a 'fresher's' hop. Freshers were first-year students, and we were encouraged to go, as it was a major 'boy meets girl' event. The invitation was not just for medical and dental students, but also for student nurses, physiotherapists, radiographers and others.

Strangely, I cannot remember whether there was live music, but feel sure there must have been. However I can remember standing with a group of fellow dental students from Blue Year, no doubt with pints of beer in our hands, surveying the girls sitting in a row along the wall on the side of the dance floor opposite us, and my eye alighted on one girl. Some of my colleagues were walking across the room and inviting the girl of their choice to dance with them, and I did not want to lose the opportunity to dance with the girl who had caught my eye.

She paused, and then got up and walked with me onto the dance floor – and we danced. As far as I can recall, we danced most of the evening. But we also talked, and I discovered that her name was Sheila, and she came from Exeter. I was a Norfolk boy, and though I had heard of Exeter and realised it was in the county of Devon in the southwest of England, had never ventured that far out of my home territory. Sheila was training to be a physiotherapist, which was not only a complete mystery to a Norfolk lad, but also rather a long word! We danced, talked a little about our families, had a drink together and danced some more. At the end of the evening I asked if we could see each other again sometime, and Sheila agreed.

* * * * * * * * * *

The studying continued, and after around ten months of preclinical training, we had an examination with a pass rate of 90%, after which 10% left the course and embarked on a different career. But before we were let loose on patients, we had first to complete the phantom head course. Wooden heads, plaster gums... but that's for another chapter.

* * * * * * * * * *

If life as a dental student at the London was proving to be a rather exciting dose of culture shock, living in Commonwealth Hall was no less so. My mother liked to remind me that I had gone to University 'to study', but I found no difficulty in reminding myself that I had come to the great metropolis to *play*. And play I did – parties till the early hours, cards through to breakfast time, and a series of self-devised practical jokes that resulted in.... well, I was thrown out! But that's for the next chapter.

CHAPTER 4

Coffee and Canasta, Wine Celebrity, and the Portly Policeman

The warden at Commonwealth Hall stared at me over the tops of his half-moon spectacles. It was to be a summary execution. "People have come to this hall to study and pass examinations, and to prepare themselves for the future. You are clearly not helping them to do this. You'll have to go. You have 24 hours notice to leave".

I had arrived at Commonwealth Hall around fourteen months earlier with an air of excitement, and anticipation of fun and fulfilment in learning how to really *live*. Life was for living, and I didn't want to miss out on it! Back in the small rural market town of North Walsham, my peers used to say that all the real life was to be found in Norwich, our local city. I felt they were the people who knew these things. But I had also met young people who actually lived in Norwich, and they had told me that all the real life was to be found in *London* – and surely these were the people who *really* knew. And so from the backwaters of rural Norfolk I had found myself in the centre of the nation's largest metropolis.

I had been shown to my room, and had unpacked my belongings, which were relatively meagre. There were tea and coffee making facilities in a small kitchen in each corridor, and having been to the nearest tobacconist and purchased a cheap packet of cigarettes, I had settled down in my armchair with a filter tip and a cup of instant coffee and pondered just how I was going to seek out this exciting city life.

In fact, I was to spend around half of my waking hours at the London studying, and that was not negotiable because I needed to pass examinations. The social life associated with the hospital and fellow students I have described in the previous chapter, but Commonwealth Hall provided me with unforgettable memories of such a wide variety of people, from all parts of the world and studying every subject imaginable. At the hospital I was rubbing shoulders with people training to be doctors and dentists, but at the hall of residence the spectrum of learning seemed almost infinite.

There were several hundred rooms at the hall, and it fairly teemed with people of every ethnicity. I soon became friendly with a number of chaps who were also on the ground floor, and my horizons started expanding. I learnt that SEES was an acronym for the School of Eastern European Studies, and one or two of my friends' courses were based there. SOAS was an acronym for the School of Oriental and African Studies, and other of my friends' were based there. Simon, who was from Norfolk, was studying nutrition, which I did not realise needed any studying, and if some of the other students' courses intrigued me, they were no less fascinated by the fact that I was training to become a dentist. "How awful", one of them said. "Why on earth do you want to be a dentist?"

I was something of a curiosity to many of them, with my Norfolk accent and naivety of the wider world. There were those from the Home Counties, who had little accent to betray their origins, who would ask, "Do you have cars in Norfolk?" and "Do you have mains drainage where you come from?" and so on. Though not poor, my parents did not have too much disposable income, and the time came when my mother decided that she would save on postage by using previously unused stamps from the collection she had built up over the years, and letters would arrive for me with the heads of long gone monarchs in the upper right hand corner of the envelope causing much mirth, and comments such as, "Hey old chap, seems the news hasn't reached Norfolk yet, but the king is dead y'know!" My mother wrote to me every week, and I enjoyed reading her letters and catching up on family news. And just occasionally we telephoned, though this was decades before mobile phones, and the small number of telephones at the hall shared between hundreds of students made using them largely impractical.

Back in Norfolk, I and my friends shared much the same degree of regional accent. The way of speaking is fairly distinctive, with the two most distinctive features being 'I' pronounced 'Oi', and words such as 'beautiful' being pronounced 'bootiful'. The mutual nature of our speech, and of most of those around us, left us largely oblivious to it. However, out of the county I found myself in very different company, not least with it being a university. The manners of many of my fellow students were impeccable, but there were those who enquired about my unusual pronunciation and intonation. I said that I did not realise that I had much of an accent, which resulted in some retorting in imitation, "Oi 'int got an accint, 'ave oi?" At times I found this embarrassing, and felt that I needed to at least 'soften' the vowels and 'firm up' the consonants if I wanted to gain credibility within the dental profession. In the latter part of the 20th century that would not have been important, but I was a student in the 1960s, and as I have explained, the culture and values within professions were different then. And so I tried to 'flatten it out', and yet half a century or so later, I am told by my wife that Norfolk intonation can still be heard if I am either tired or angry. And of course, when I returned to Norfolk during University holidays, my local friends would ask, "Why are you speaking like *that*?"

But it was the different personalities that I enjoyed so much. Richard Rankin had done some preliminary training at Cambridge prior to arriving in London to study medicine at St. Thomas' Hospital, but was (almost) a professional entertainer. He was 'frightfully public school', called people 'old man', and had teamed up with another medic as a comedy duo performing cabaret at some of the more upmarket West End clubs. Coffee with Richard had more than a touch of cabaret about it too. Anthony Graham Hipson-Ruth Smith from Oxford wore a monocle, had appeared on the television programme University Challenge, and was rumoured to have an IQ off the end of the scale. No-one seemed to know what he was studying – or maybe no-one could understand. He played strange war games, where other residents were assigned countries, armies, navies, etc. and engaged one another in furtive conversations around the more shadowy corridors of the hall. I introduced myself to him, was included in a game and soon annihilated. The beturbanned Professor Shan hailed from the Punjab, was studying philosophy of some description, and enjoyed showing me photographs of his wife and children, and was eagerly looking forward to being reunited with them. "Please come and visit us one day", he said warmly. Mr. Gann (he was always known as 'Mr. Gann') came from the People's Republic of China, and seemed somewhat aloof and separate from the rest of us. Did anyone get to know Mr. Gann? My closer friends were engaged in more conventional studies such as mathematics (Dave – who seemed to have around three lectures a week and a photographic memory that ensured he had the rest of the time at leisure), Russian (Trevor, known for some reason as 'Fritz'), and English (another Dave, who talked a lot about the Boys Brigade which had been an important part of his younger life, and who drowned in a swimming pool in Switzerland during the summer at the end of our first year). Dave, who studied Maths, had come back to my home in Norfolk for a weekend, and my sister appeared quite smitten with the chap. But girls to Dave were like bees round a honey-pot – what is it about some fellows? And Fritz joined me on a cottage holiday in the wilds of north Wales where, together with a fellow dental student, we combed the bars of Abersoch in search of French au pair girls – and found a few!

These months at Commonwealth Hall were times of great discovery, and one of the greatest was that of Indian food.

Opposite the hall was a restaurant, with the word 'Bengal' in its name, and I felt attracted like an iron filing to a powerful magnet. I was not disappointed, and felt I had come close to finding heaven on earth (though that was really to come later). Indian food has been an integral part of my life since that first visit in 1963.

* * * * * * * * * *

'Norfolk boy has unusual taste for fine wines' read the headline for an article in a local paper a few months after I had left for London, and continued to describe how the young man had also an exquisite knowledge of sherry production and of the different types. As usual, my name was spelt incorrectly as Barry, and not Barrie, but the photograph was clearly the local lad, once of 'mousing' fame, and now training to be a dentist at the London.

I had never drunk a glass of wine in my life before going to London a few months earlier, and as for sherry, that was something only my *grandmother* drank. My parents imbibed tea almost exclusively, and life at the London had introduced me to beer, but when a flier appeared on the notice board at Commonwealth Hall advertising a meeting of the University Wine and Food Society, I felt a deep attraction. Here was my opportunity, not only to gain knowledge of wines and foods of distinction (though quite frankly any wines and foods would have been acceptable), but also the almost certain consumption of vast quantities of both. To a student on a very modest grant, the kudos ('fine wine' and 'gourmet' food) and the plain animal satisfaction of imbibing and consuming, was irresistible.

A number of medical students were present at the meeting (their fathers were consultants and they mainly preferred 'the red stuff'), as well as several well-spoken chaps from other disciplines – and me. Containers filled with sawdust were there for spitting wine into, but appeared to be bone dry at the end of the meeting. When newcomers were invited to 'sign up',

I could just about focus my eyes sufficiently to scrawl my name on the dotted line. That's about all I can remember of that first meeting, but I left it as a 'member'.

It was only a month or two later that the 'University Sherry Competition' was announced. It took the form of an essay on the subject of 'Sherry', and the judge was to be an acclaimed authority (his name escapes me) on the stuff, and who had written a series of advertisements for a sherry producer (whose name escapes me again), which was appearing every weekend in the quality colour supplements at that time. Newspapers were supplied to the common rooms at Commonwealth Hall, and I lost no time in seeking out the advertisements. They were beautiful, each one designed to appear as a parchment unfurled across the page, and each of the series of six described some aspect of sherry –its history, its production, the different types, and so on. This was way beyond my knowledge until..... it seemed such a silly idea, but appealed to my sense of humour and that of some of my friends at the hall. I collected the series of six advertisements, and sat down to rewrite them, almost word for word, but with a different order of paragraphs where the sense of the passage was not overly compromised, and after just an evening, had devised an entry.

It was with some trepidation that I attended the meeting of the Wine and Food Society at which the great man himself was to announce the winner of the competition, and I wondered whether he might make some rather critical comments about an idiot entry he had come across. Having announced the runners up, I could hardly believe my ears, or yet contain myself, when he proclaimed me the winner, and spoke of my comprehensive knowledge and clarity of communication on the subject of sherry. I was awarded several bottles of sherry, a glass vessel used by professional tasters, and a silver 'venencia' like those used to draw sherry from the butts during the production process in Spain. And, of course, I was now fêted as a previously unrecognised celebrity amongst my peers within the Society.

A month or so later, the annual 'University Wine Tasting Competition' was announced, and I was enthusiastically encouraged to represent the Society. I cannot remember who was eligible to enter, or who competed against whom, but I was in a team of four, and we were to taste, identify and make comments on six wines, of which three would be red burgundies, and three clarets. I was a complete novice, not really knowing what a 'claret' or a 'burgundy' was or where it came from. However, I had some coaching before the competition, and I started to grasp something of the nature of the red wines from these two different regions of France. I was also given some other useful advice from our coach, namely that the man who was to judge the tasting was also the one who would supply the wine – and he was known to be incredibly mean. So why was he supplying free wine for the competition? – in order to get publicity and promote sales. And what would the wine be like? – cheap and definitely non-vintage. The vintage of a wine refers to the year of its production, and gives some indication of the quality of the wine. Left over wine from different years from a region can be mixed together and bottled up, but does not have a vintage. Well, it could be anything! The relevance of this information was that I would have to answer three questions, and then give 'further comments', and here was an opportunity to pick up points. By writing 'non-vintage' in the comments column for each wine, I was told I was assured of getting five points out of a possible six.

The evening arrived, and I duly sniffed and gurgled each of the six wines in turn, spitting and rinsing between glasses. And our team came second, out of quite a number of entrants. I had been successful in identifying the burgundies and the clarets, and some of the regions. And under the 'Comments' section I picked up five additional points, which was a great contribution to the team's score.

At the end of that academic year the Wine and Food Society met to elect officers for the coming year, and my name was one of the first put forward. I really felt totally inadequate to take much responsibility, not least because of the demanding nature of the dental course and the rest of my social life, and so I simply became a committee member. I soon discovered that I now had certain material advantages over the ordinary members.

A typical Wine and Food Society evening would centre upon studying, say, the wines of the Loire. The evening would start with the arrival of the committee in time to take delivery of the wines, donated by a merchant who hoped that the credit for his donation would result in later sales. Several cases would be delivered, and the committee's first task was to hide a few. The speaker would arrive, and then the members of the Society. The speaker would cover his subject, Wines of the Loire, describing their history, production, variety and distinctive features, while the members fidgeted impatiently. Corks were drawn, glasses filled, and wines 'tasted' with enthusiasm. Pots of sawdust remained as dry as they had at the start, and when the bottles were empty, the speaker was thanked, the next meeting announced, and the members would depart. The doors were then closed and the hidden cases brought out for distribution among the committee members, who would make their way home to their respective halls, flats, or wherever.

We also had an annual dinner with a celebrity (real celebrity!) speaker, and those of us on the committee would enjoy his company for pre-dinner drinks. I shall always remember the evening a few of us sat with Clement Freud, a man of dry wit, active mind, and a real knowledge of wine and food. Maybe my account of the Society is just a little tongue in cheek, though there was certainly more than a degree of the sort of student over-indulgence that one would reasonably expect in such company. I learned quite a lot about wine in those days, though little about food, and have enjoyed wine, and some especially, most of my life since.

* * * * * * * * * *

And then there was Sheila, my first university girlfriend. We arranged to meet again, though I cannot remember where, or what we did. I would not be surprised if she can though, because that is the way ladies are made. But she came round to Commonwealth Hall for evening dinner on a few occasions, and we would sometimes simply walk and talk. Our conversations covered all the usual boy/girl topics, including family, history, hopes and dreams, and.... religion. And here was our problem, for whereas Sheila was a practising and convinced Christian, I was an atheist (who went to church, mainly because my grandfather, for whom I had immense respect, had asked me to 'go to church.' But it was an *occasional* practice only).

I had been an atheist since my early teenage years. Our family had not gone to church when I was a child, and when I was taught evolution at grammar school, I could in no way reconcile that with my concept of the God of the Bible, and I stated quite unequivocally that I was an atheist. A few years after this we had moved to a town where there was a church of my mother's denomination and as a family we had attended on Sundays. But I would not become a 'member', even when the rest of the family did, and continued to declare myself an atheist, finding comfort in the fact that the choir master said that he was an atheist too. And I suspected that many others in the elderly congregation were not at all sure themselves.

But Sheila was sure, and we debated this at length. How could there be a God when there was so much suffering in the world, I argued, and she told me that mankind was responsible for most of the suffering. How could she reconcile the creation story with science, was another question I had, and she told me that many scientists were in fact believers. We talked about the fact that there were so many religions, and I wanted to know how she could be certain that Christianity was right and all the others wrong. She then argued that the one true God created all things, and that people, having separated themselves from this God, developed their own faiths and religions to satisfy their need of one. Christ had made a way back to the true God, she explained.

I enjoyed debating these things, and part of student life has always been to put the world right by debating politics and religion. Sheila and I were fond of each other, but I could not persuade her that atheism was true, and she could not convince me that the God of the Bible was real. She explained to me that for a believer to partner a non-believer had all sorts of practical, as well as Biblical, problems, and felt it best that we stop seeing each other in view of the fact that there could be no future for us. And so we parted company.

But those days had been special, and I had a lot of respect for Sheila, her faith and her principles. I went on to take a number of other ladies out, but had precious memories of those times with Sheila. On several occasions I had taken her back to her Hall of Residence, John Harrison House in Whitechapel, and in doing so had missed the last underground train back to Bloomsbury, and walked the five miles or so through east London, arriving back in the early hours of the morning.

* * * * * * * * * *

"You have 24 hours from now to leave this hall," said the warden. It would be unthinkable for that to happen today, and was deemed to be a harsh judgement in those days too.

I had always been fascinated with practical jokes, and at school had doctored the chalk so that it exploded when drawn across the blackboard. It was just cordite from the 'caps' used in toy pistols, but it left the smell of gunfire in the air and sent the maths master trembling back to the staff room. Elephant traps had fascinated me, but there was no opportunity, and buckets of water over doors had seemed almost irresistible – yet I had never had the nerve. But now I was at university, and found at last a freedom of expression in this aspect of life and interest – but it led to my ejection from Commonwealth Hall!

During that first year at the hall much of the social life was getting to know new people, and sitting and chatting over coffee, often until the early hours. Most of us smoked, and most of us drank beer, and wine was of course making its way onto the scene. A number of us found that we had the card game canasta in common and would sit up and play until late.

At the end of each year at the hall there was a reallocation of rooms, and in September 1964 I found myself in a room on the front of the hall on the seventh floor. Late in the evening friends would come round for coffee (why did *my* room so often be the meeting place?) and we often got out two packs of playing cards and ended up playing canasta until the early hours, with the odd break for coffee and a cigarette. But I had an idea for entertainment of a different kind.

I took a tin lid to the hospital, and used my dental drill to make a hole in it, and then purchased a reel of black cotton. I tied the tin lid to the cotton, and the next time my friends came round, I had something to show them! It was around 3 a.m. during one of our coffee breaks, and I drew back the curtains and opened the window. My seventh floor window opened out onto Cartwright Gardens, and we could hear the distant rumble of traffic on Tottenham Court Road, though there was significantly less in those days, especially during the small hours of the morning. We peered down, and saw that almost every other light was off, and the students no doubt sleeping. I lowered the tin lid until it was level with the second floor windows, and then proceeded to swing it, covering around a dozen or more windows from that height. And then I pulled it in sharply, and it rattled along the length of the windows. And then back again, after which I pulled it up a storey or two, had someone turn my room light off, and we waited and watched.

Sure enough, lights started to go on along the second floor, and then we could see curtains being drawn back as light shone out from closed windows. Closed – but not for long, and suddenly it seemed that all along the second floor, windows were opening and heads unlike any I had seen in Norfolk emerged and – peered down! The novelty of seeing so many people of other ethnicities had still not worn off for this Norfolk boy, and certain floors in Commonwealth Hall were occupied largely by communities from different parts of our former empire. Who had knocked on their windows? Each then realised that they were not alone in having someone rap on their window, and from staring down two floors, they started talking to each other in languages that were certainly foreign to me and my companions. And then, one by one, the heads would be withdrawn, windows close, curtains drawn and the lights would go out. Which was the cue for rapping on a further dozen or more windows – on the third floor.

We did not do this too often, but it appealed to our callous sense of humour to give our 'foreign friends' a wake-up call from time to time. It was not racism, as we did not know that floor was occupied largely by Africans until the first night that the heads came out, and we would have proceeded regardless of ethnicity. And then one night, someone looked up instead of down. And that was the final night of the tin lid.

I felt that there was more scope for my creativity in this area of entertainment, and one evening had what I considered a brainwave. The outside and inside handles of each room door are connected by an internal 'communicating rod', for which there is probably a technical name. This rod is itself connected to the metal nib (or catch) that fits into the hole in the doorpost. By turning the door handle(s) the rod twists and withdraws the metal nib from the hole. Hey presto, the door opens! After experimenting on my own door, I was ready for action.

Girls were allowed in resident's rooms, but had to be signed in, and signed out again by 10 p.m. I and my friends decided upon the victim, and waited for him to take his girlfriend into his room and lock the door. Soon we could hear music playing, which was really necessary for what I had in mind. I carefully and quietly unscrewed the plate that held the door handle in place, and after removing it and exposing the communicating rod, removed that too. I then quietly replaced the outer door handle. At about twenty minutes to ten, we knocked loudly on the door, and then waited. After a minute or two of regaining their composure, we could hear the inner door handle being turned – but to no avail. There were no telephones in the rooms, and the mobile phone had not been invented, and after a while the unfortunate man would give up. At this point I would slip the rod back into the door, and we would run. The student and his girlfriend would fairly sprint to the lift and down to reception, embarrassingly explaining that the door had jammed. Of course, the outer plate had to be screwed back in place, and this was done while the student was making his exit downstairs.

But I realised that my identity as the culprit would not remain concealed forever, and so took precautions for the evening when it would happen to me. There was a laundry room on each floor, with washing machines and clothes lines, and with wooden slatting on the floor to prevent the launderers getting their feet wet from the water dripping in steady streams from the array of laundered garments. I crept along to one with my screwdriver, and after removing the communicating rod from the door, propped it open with a wooden wedge. It was not too long before, whilst entertaining a guest of the female variety, I detected some tell-tale sounds from the area of my door handle. Around a quarter to ten, I removed the plate and handle from the inside of my door (girlfriend looking on in astonishment), inserted the rod, and flung open the door, in time to see amazed residents, indeed those I considered my friends and fellow conspirators, dashing away along the corridor. But there was an unfortunate sequel.

The laundry room from which I had removed the rod was on a different floor from my own, and one mainly occupied by Oriental students, one of whom decided to launder during the small hours of the morning. Being a considerate gentleman, he removed the wedge from the door and closed the door in order to keep the noise from disturbing his fellows. Needless to say, he spent the night sleeping on the slats, and was rescued by a handyman the following day, when his plight was made known.

"You have 24 hours from now to leave this hall," said the warden. I felt that being given a warning would have been more appropriate, but the warden had made up his mind. Twenty-four hours – that really left me in a dreadful dilemma, and fortunately I was not alone in feeling that this was a case of overkill. A number of other residents quickly rushed round with a petition requesting that I be allowed to stay in the Hall, and as a result I was given until the end of the term.

There was a waiting list for rooms at the Students Hostel that was part of the hospital complex in Whitechapel, but I went and saw those who administered the hostel, and after explaining my situation, was given a room there immediately. I was amazed at this, and felt that there would be a string of conditions attached, but this was not the case. And when I moved in and experienced life there amongst my fellow dental students and medics, I realised that any pranks I had engaged in at Commonwealth Hall were really quite tame compared with some of the happenings at the Students Hostel.

I had enjoyed my time at Commonwealth Hall, and it had contributed immensely to my education. The friends I had made, of various ethnicities, of differing degree courses and with great personalities, will live on in my memory forever. But it was 'goodbye' to Commonwealth Hall, and after some time, I lost touch with most of those I had been so close to. But there was one more memorable incident involving Commonwealth Hall before I move on.

* * * * * * * * * *

I received a message from some of my friends back at Cartwright Gardens that they were going to a party one evening, and enquired whether I would like to join them. They would be driving, as one of their number had a car. I would be welcome to join them, but by the time we got back to the Hall, the Underground trains would have stopped running and I would be obliged to make my own arrangements for getting back to Whitechapel. By this time I had my bicycle in London, and so I cycled over to Bloomsbury, went to the party in their car, and arrived back at the Hall there at around 4 a.m. I tried to sit on the bicycle, but my vision was at least double, and my balance non-existent. That was the nature of the parties we went to, and that was the nature of Barrie. So my friends helped me onto the bike, and gave me a push in the direction of Whitechapel, which was around five miles away.

London traffic was reasonably light at night in those days, and I coped quite well until I came to a junction of five roads in that part of London known as 'the City' or in Underground terms, 'Bank'. The traffic light was red, and I stopped. I was wobbling a lot, and trying not to fall over, standing astride the bicycle. Instead of watching the light for my road, I decided to watch the green light of one of the other roads that was visible from where I stood, and when it went red, and forgetting that there were five roads and not a simple crossroads, I started lurching on the bike, pedaling wildly across the junction.

How could such a large policeman be so invisible? With my vision in the state it was, I should have seen him - twice! Slowly he stepped off the dimly-lit traffic island in the centre of the junction, and shone his torch at me. "OK you," he said in typical police fashion. "Get off that bike!" I suppose we all make strange and unaccountable decisions at times in our lives, and sometimes they can lead to disastrous consequences that cannot easily be undone, if at all. It was a split second decision, but inexplicably, I lowered my head and cycled at him for all I was worth. I saw his eyes open wide as a look of alarm flashed across his face, and suddenly the portly policeman was no longer in my way, but had fairly leapt back onto the traffic island. Behind me now were shouts of "Hey you, come back 'ere" and "Get off that bike" and something about "the law", but with heart pounding I cycled like the proverbial 'bat out of hell', taking a right turn, then a left, then another left, then a right and so on, determined to shake off and totally confuse any pursuer. Back at the Students Hostel, I carried my bike down to the basement, hid it under the billiard table, raced to my room and having locked the door, laid on my bed with the light out and waited for the plod of police feet – which never came of course.

Maybe I was making up for a somewhat straitened lifestyle at home, where study, study, study had taken up such a lot of my life. But my health was starting to suffer, and if I was ever to become a professional gentleman in a white coat, there was a lot of work to be done.

Unbeknown to me however, some big changes to my life were just around the corner.

CHAPTER 5

Phantom Heads, a Five-Hour Filling, and the Damascus Road

"Can you remember doing your first filling?" I've been asked on a few occasions. "Yes - and I'm sure the patient can too!" I reply. That I shall come to shortly.

Carrying out ones first filling was quite an experience for both the student and the unsuspecting (but probably not for long) patient, and so in those days, we had an intensive course of practising on 'phantom heads' first. Let me take you into the 'Phantom Head' room. We enter a long narrow room through a door in one of the narrow walls, and find that there are work tops running the length of both the opposing long walls. At intervals of around four feet, wooden heads are bolted to the work surface, and they are facing the wall. Each head has hinged brass jaws, and set into plaster of Paris gums are plastic teeth. By each head there is a stool, and hanging from the ceiling, and alongside each head, is a drill. On the wall at the end of the room is mounted a blackboard. A student sits on each stool, poised over the head with a mouth mirror in his left hand and a drill in his right.

"OK chaps," says the tutor, standing by the blackboard. He works part time at the London and part time in his practice in Harley Street, and the lesser staff and students at the hospital whisper to one another, "He has a practice in Harley Street, you know" and his patients in Harley Street confide in each other, "He trains student dentists at a big teaching hospital, you know." The tutor continues, "Place your drill on the centre of the surface of the tooth, and gently - and I mean *gently* - go down through the surface enamel, until it plops into the cavity." He continues to describe how to remove the decay (we had to call it 'caries') and of the most desirable shape of filling cavity (we had to call it 'outline form'). And then we had to proceed to fill a tooth on the phantom head, using only the 'slow drill' as we were deemed too inexperienced to use the newer 'fast' air-driven turbines. We had to learn to live in an upside down world viewed through the mouth mirror, and we had to learn *not* to clear the plastic dust that accumulated with a sharp blow from our mouth!

Have you heard your dentist use the expression MO, DO, or MOD? In general terms the front surface of a tooth is referred to by dentists as the mesial, the back as the distal, and the biting surface the occlusal, and cavities and fillings are abbreviated to denote the surfaces involved. Permanent teeth are denoted by numerals from 1 to 8, where 1 is the central incisor at the front, and 8 is the wisdom tooth. Upper left, lower right and so on completes the tooth's description, such as upper right 4, or lower left 6. Deciduous ('baby') teeth are denoted A to E, and the most difficult filling was deemed to be an MO on an upper left 4, and that was the filling we had to do after three months of drilling and filling on these phantom heads. We all passed a week or two before Christmas 1964 (though I had to do mine twice in order to convince the examiner) and then had a short break before returning to spend the next four years working on live patients.

* * * * * * * * *

Most of us were going to work in general practice, and would be looking after people's teeth, gums and gaps from the cradle to the grave. So patients of all ages and types were assigned to each of us, and we were responsible for their dental health for the duration of our training. There were adults, children and teenagers, with all their teeth, or some of their teeth, or none of their teeth. Some had straight teeth, and some crooked; some had healthy gums, and some were grossly infected; some were relaxed, and others were understandably nervous. We examined teeth and gums, and carried out fillings, extractions, crowns, and bridges; crooked teeth were straightened; infected gums were made healthy, often through surgery (we cut the infected gums away). We constructed partial and full dentures, and fitted them in the clinics. We were watched like hawks in our early days, and every item of treatment had to be checked at every stage. The days were taken up with working in clinics (patients) and laboratories (crowns and dentures) and we also had several lectures a week. The hospital even managed to squeeze in one year of medicine, surgery, pathology, etc. for us, and in the evenings most of us needed to study at length. And there were parties, and canasta; and as Easter approached in 1965, I started suffering from stress (*and* was told to find new accommodation!).

"Today you will each carry out your first filling on a real patient," said the tutor. Some of Blue Year looked quite calm and professional, whereas others looked positively excited. I was terrified. Suppose the cavity was at the back of the mouth and the patient choked, or suppose the cavity was anywhere - and the patient choked? Suppose I skidded into the gum? My mind was full of negative thoughts as we were each led off to a dental chair, where our respective patients were waiting. They had already had their injection to numb the tooth.

"Mr. Lawrence - this lady needs a filling here in the front of her upper left 1. Quite simple, old chap. I'll leave you to it."

I introduced myself, and the patient leant back in the chair and opened her mouth. I gingerly touched the tooth with the drill, barely tickling it, and withdrew. Hardly a mark. I repeated the procedure, with the same non-result, and offered the patient a rinse. The decay was small and the enamel hard, and when I pressed a bit harder, the drill skidded, and the cavity got wider. This continued for around three hours, with intermittent rinses, after which it was time for the clinic to close for the day. I tried to put a temporary dressing in the cavity, but though it was wide, in fact very wide, it was not sufficiently deep to retain a dressing, which kept falling out. And so the patient went home, and I went to the Sammie for a pint with the rest of Blue Year.

It was three weeks later when the patient returned, and after a further two hours, it was finished. Much of the front of the lady's tooth was now a large, roughly circular cavity. I was concerned about making it look too dark, and countered this by selecting the whitest filling material I could find. As the patient left the clinic she smiled broadly, and the filling appeared like a large headlight beaming out of her mouth and showing her the way home!

We spent hours and hours in that clinic, and some of those early days were more than a little fraught. Sometimes we had to practise on one another, and soon learnt who to avoid. Henry Levine was known as 'danger man' - but not to his face. He was thorough, fast, silent, and deadly. He worked with great panache - but was accident prone. Our dental chairs were constructed of cast iron and were known as 'sit up and beg' chairs. They weighed a ton, and once the patient was seated, would be tipped back and secured with a small lever located by the dentist's right foot. When treatment was complete, the dentist would hold the chair firmly whilst releasing the foot lever, and the weight of chair and patient would tip it forward to its starting position. Henry would tip the patient back, swing round to pick up his mirror and probe, and inadvertently rest his foot on the release lever. CRASH - a ton of cast iron chair would lurch forward, the patient rapidly gaining velocity and about to be propelled across the clinic when Henry would fling his arms round the patient and save them from serious injury. Heads would look up around the clinic, and the words 'Henry!' and 'Danger Man' would be muttered, and knowing winks exchanged. During scaling sessions, several of Henry's patients actually fainted, possibly encouraged by the student himself saying sternly "We have to be cruel to be kind here." Some of his patients looked as though they had been involved in road traffic accidents, but it was simply blood from that enthusiastic scaling technique, which also resulted in more than a few crowns 'popping off'', with the gold ones apparently landing in his pocket. What became of Henry? The last time I saw him he was a consultant.

But it was not just some of the students who were given a wide berth. A new registrar arrived at the hospital to work in the Oral Surgery (extractions) department. He was a huge rough looking fellow, generally described as half Neanderthal and half gorilla, and his reputation as such was forever sealed when a patient attending to have a tooth extracted took one look at him and passed out. Quick as lightning he grabbed some nearby forceps, knelt beside the patient and opening their mouth, had the tooth out before anyone had a chance to realise what was happening. The patient gave a shout and jumped up, and was led away by a nurse to the recovery area. "Seize the moment," championed the gorilla. "The tooth is out, the patient has been brought round from their faint, and all without having to give an injection." Today there would be disciplinary hearings, suspension, litigation......

Ron liked to have a beaker of cold water at his side. The canteen was some distance away, the clinic could get warm, and Ron would get thirsty. Ron also had a beaker of water in which patients, having removed their dentures from their somewhat foody, debris-strewn mouths, would place their false teeth. One day, after such a patient had left, Ron, being thirsty, drank the beaker of water, and as he swallowed it, detected lots of little pieces....... Wrong beaker!

Rob had spent hours and hours setting up the trial dentures for a patient. They were made basically of pink wax, in which were set the plastic teeth that would be used in the final, processed set of dentures. They appeared to fit correctly, met together properly, and the patient liked the appearance of them. But Rob had to have the work inspected at this stage, and went to get a member of staff to have a look and give the required signature. The member of staff was explaining a procedure to another student, and a further two or three were waiting, and when Rob returned to his patient, the chair was empty and the wax dentures were gone. One floor below, in the patient's cafeteria, the man who had walked in with a pristine smile and ordered a hot cup of tea, was to be seen removing a huge sticky lump of pink wax from his mouth, with plastic teeth protruding at all angles. Hot tea melts wax!

I can vividly remember giving my first injection, and like my first filling, I'm sure the patient can clearly remember it too. Half of Blue Year was taken to a large surgery where they were each to carry out their first extraction, while the other half of us were taken to another surgery where we were to give the injections to numb the teeth to be extracted. It was my turn, and the consultant briefed me. "It's an upper molar to be extracted. Penetrate the gum on the outside of the tooth. It's soft and you can glide your needle up into the tissues and deposit the anaesthetic. Now, the roof of the mouth is different. It's fibrous and tough, and its bound tightly to the bony palate, so you'll have to go in quite hard. Don't be afraid of it, and make sure you reach the bone."

My patient entered the surgery, and was probably the largest Negress I had ever set eyes on. Even her name was huge, and seemed to incorporate a lot of Old Testament Bible names, ending in Abraham. I'm not sure whether she sat in the chair, on the chair, or over the chair, and I had to lean a long way to even see the tooth. I penetrated the soft outside gum tissues and deposited the anaesthetic. "OK?" asked the consultant, and I nodded. The syringe was refilled with anaesthetic solution, and I leaned forward and took aim at the roof of the mouth, just in from the offending molar. Pow - I indeed 'went in quite hard', but hardly had the needle penetrated the fibrous tissue and hit the underlying bone, than the patient gave a shout, rose in the chair, and in doing so extricated herself from the needle, which was now hovering just above the tongue. On the roof of the mouth was a small bleeding dot-like lesion. "OK?" asked the consultant, and I shook my head silently. "Come on man," he said in a low voice, and I again took aim and plunged the needle into the roof of the mouth. As it hit the bone, there was another shout from the patient, and as she jumped out from the needle, I noticed there were now two little bleeding spots on the roof of the mouth. The consultant was breathing down the back of my neck as he asked rather shortly, "OK now?" I explained that it was not, and he rather impatiently told me to 'get on with it', and again I took aim and plunged in the syringe. There was another shout and another bleeding dot, and again the consultant asked, "OK now?" I had had enough, as had the patient, and at that time in my life was not averse to telling a little white lie now and again. I nodded, and in response the consultant indicated I should press the plunger home and deliver the anaesthetic. It came out of the end of the needle like a fountain, dripped off the upper teeth, and formed a puddle under the tongue. "Can I spit?" asked the patiently, understandably, only to have the consultant respond with "No dear - swallow." She pulled a face that matched the taste of the anaesthetic she swallowed, and was ushered out of the surgery and along to my colleagues who were waiting to extract the molar. They didn't, because the tooth was not numb. And nor were half the injected teeth that day, but all the failures were then anaesthetised by the consultant, and had their teeth extracted by another consultant. They were considered to have suffered enough.

And I went off to the Sammie with the rest of Blue Year, because I thought that I had suffered enough too that day!

* * * * * * * * * *

I have extracted, if you'll forgive the pun, some of those moments that I find memorable in being humorous or poignant. But most of the course was hard work, with the days being demanding in terms of the intensive nature of dental training. I have always felt privileged to be a part of Blue Year, and most of my patients were decent people, keen to help me in any way they could, and grateful for the treatment they received. But as I wrote in an earlier chapter, I am of mediocre ability academically, and needed my evenings for studying. Partying, staying up until the early hours playing cards and so forth, was more than I could comfortably cope with, and I started suffering with stress. I became quite tense and found relating to people, and conversations in general, increasingly difficult. Being told to change my accommodation had added another stress factor to my life and the hospital doctor prescribed Librium, which might have helped but is difficult to evaluate.

I was now living at the Students Hostel, virtually attached to the hospital itself, and not long after moving there met Sheila again. She continued to live at John Harrison House, a stone's throw from the hostel, and we would often stop and chat briefly on our way to our respective studies.

She was concerned at the stress symptoms that I was suffering, and we would from time to time get onto the subject of her Christian faith. With hindsight, it was no coincidence that a number of other 'born again' Christians crossed my path at this time.

Christians! There were quite a few around, and I just could not understand them. I enjoyed their company, usually, but could not understand their faith, ever. Almost everything I had been taught at school, read in books and newspapers, seen on the television, and so on, seemed to assume that we were upmarket *animals*, the ultimate product of a process known as evolution. But the Christians I met had a very different world view, and asserted that we had been created, and that their lives had been changed by the Creator. And when they had to admit to me that only those people who had been 'born again' would be spending eternity with this Creator God......... arrogant bigots! And yet they were not. They were intelligent people training to be doctors, nurses, physiotherapists, and in one case, a dentist. They were caring and had warm personalities, and I felt they were not primarily trying to win an argument, but wanting to help me.

How did I meet them? They were lurking everywhere, so it seemed. I couldn't help overhearing conversations in our athenaeum (men's common room) at the hostel, which was a useful thing to do as one could pick up good jokes, or learn where the cheapest beer could be found. However, on some occasions the conversation overheard would be of a problem 'being prayed about' or 'but what does the Bible say?', and I realised that the God Squad was around. They fascinated me, and I would introduce myself and enquire whether I could ask a question. "Fire away," they would say, and I would give them evolution, different faiths, the problem of suffering, and so on. They didn't always have the answers, but I liked the people.

Life in the hostel was a lot different from that in the University hall. It was much smaller, and we were all studying medicine or dentistry. There were maybe a hundred students, of whom about ten were ladies, who had their own corridor. They kept themselves to themselves, and were not allowed in the athenaeum. Most definitely not! A minority of students were rowdy, often drunk, and occasionally violent. I have no doubt that many of them had distinguished careers and are now retired doctors. Many were gifted sportsmen and several played rugby for the hospital. It was said that they could fail as many exams as they liked, but as long as they did well for the hospital on the rugby field, they were safe. There was also a rumour that in earlier years prospective medical students attending for interview would find that, on entering the interview room, the dean would lob a piece of crumpled paper at them. If the student instinctively caught it, or alternatively kicked or headed it into the waste paper bin, he was in. If he jumped to one side, or fumbled it, he was turned down.

I explored the area around the hospital and hostel. Rows and rows of Victorian terraced houses with basement flats, contrasted with the modern architecture of the hospital, which was continually expanding. Streets would vanish, and new laboratories or research buildings were always appearing. The docks were less than a half hour walk away, at Wapping where the Thames looked particularly grubby. There were a few Indian restaurants, and it was at one on Whitechapel Road that I was to have my first vindaloo. I bragged about it for weeks!

There was a hairdresser with a most unusual illuminated sign. These days, I would not let such a photo opportunity pass, but in those days I had a primitive camera that used expensive films which needed expensive processing. Expensive for a student, that is. The sign? A Greek Cypriot named Christopher had settled in the area and decided to set up as a hairdresser. He went to a fellow Greek Cypriot who was a maker of illuminated signs, and told him what he wanted. The sign maker explained to Christopher that in England his name was shortened - but he wasn't sure quite how short the name was. The result - an illuminated sign which boldly declared CHRIST'S HAIRDRESSER. I couldn't believe it when I first saw it, and assumed it would not be there for long. However, it was there throughout my Whitechapel years, but vanished together with the rest of the street some years later to make room for, you guessed it, another extension of the hospital.

And so it seemed that I could not get away from Christ, as he was spoken of from the hostel athenaeum to the local Cypriot hairdresser. I was not sure whether I wanted to 'get away' from the subject, but I *did* want to know whether it was true. If God is real, I needed to know. In fact, we each need to know. *Need* to know, because if the Bible is true, there will come a day when we stand before him. *Need* to know, because he promises 'abundant life', which in everyday English means a fulfilled life that nothing else can give us.

The Christians I met said they *knew* him, and though I had conversed with a number of Hindus, Jews, Buddhists and members of just about every other religion during my days at Commonwealth Hall, only Christians really *knew* God. If they did. So I started sending up the occasional 'Are you there?' prayer, and read some of the Gospel stories of Jesus. I also read some other parts of the Bible, including the account of Saul on the road to Damascus having a dramatic conversion experience. I felt it would take a similar encounter with Christ to convert me, but I realised that it was an all-or-nothing business; if God was real, and if Christ had died to demolish the 'sin barrier' that prevents us knowing God until we come properly to accept him, then I would give him my all. On the other hand, if I found he was not there (I felt that was a probability), then he would of course get nothing from me.

And one day, sitting in my room at the hostel, I sensed the presence of God. This was something altogether new, and almost scared me. How had it happened? How should I respond? I had certainly been seeking the truth concerning these things, and I had read something Jesus had said about 'those who seek will find', but I found it a little difficult to come to terms with my new 'faith'. Did this make me a Christian? Was I now a member of the God Squad? But I could not get away from the fact that there was a presence in my life that had never ever been there before, and I knew who he was.

Life goes on, and I continued drilling and filling, injecting and extracting, and all the time feeling rather smug because I now knew something that most people did not seem to know. And in my heart, I was an arrogant bigot!

It must have been about a month later, in October 1965 shortly after my 21st birthday, that I suddenly realised that, if I now knew the God of the Bible to be real - and I did, and he was - then I needed to respond to that knowledge. And although it sounds awfully pious and might even cause some to cringe, in the early hours of one morning that October, having finished studying for the evening, I knelt down on the floor of my hostel room, and prayed, thanking God for revealing himself to me, thanking him for Jesus, giving myself to him to serve in any way called, and asking for his strength to do so. And then I went to bed.

The next morning I got up, thought back to the previous night, and realised that I felt different. How? Different inside.

A sense of security. A sense of fulfilment. 'Joy' sounds like a cliché, but comes close to describing it. And that was the end of Barrie taking Librium!

So Barrie had indeed had a Damascus Road experience, though it had all taken a bit longer than that of Paul the apostle. Life went on, with teeth always on the agenda and romance in the air, though I did not quite realise it at the time. And as everything seemed to be a little different now, with everything seen in a new light, somehow holey teeth had become holy teeth!

CHAPTER 6

The 'Und Here Syndrome', a Sapphire Ring, and a Monkey with a Pistol

"Und Here Syndrome" was written quite clearly across the top of Mrs. Bergstein's dental records. But I had never heard of this condition before. Might it render her allergic to the dental anaesthetic I was about to use, or might she need to take antibiotics before I extracted a tooth? I racked my brains. I had already completed a course of medicine, surgery, pathology, bacteriology, pharmacology and therapeutics, and though there would always be some obscure diseases I would never know about, this was written quite clearly on the notes, as though *everybody* knew what the Und Here Syndrome was.

I told the patient I would be back shortly and found one of the dental tutors.

"What's the Und Here Syndrome?" I asked. He gave a broad smile, and said, "Read further down."

I did so and read the words "Jewish Complaining type." I must have looked a little blank at this too, because the tutor continued, using an accent that I could only describe as roughly 'Continental'-

"Doctor, I haff a pain, here...... und here..... und here... und here..."

Poor Mrs. Bergstein. She suffered most of her life from the Und Here Syndrome, which was a recognized condition of a small minority of the Jewish patients we had at the hospital, and might best be described as a form of hypochondria. Apparently there was quite a lot of it about at times.

Another Jewish patient, Solomon Godfrey, asked me if I had a girlfriend, and when I answered in the affirmative, responded with, "Then bring me her measurements, my boy."

"Why should I?" I exclaimed, to be greeted with a broad grin and the explanation, "Because I am a tailor, and will make her a sexy skirt for you."

So I asked Sheila for a few measurements, and a fortnight later she had a grey miniskirt to parade around in. Well, around the flat she had moved into, and not much beyond its confines!

Mrs. Stuart was a plumpish pleasant middle-aged lady from one of the north-eastern suburbs called Redbridge. Typically, when a small businessman in Whitechapel did well for himself, he moved on to Redbridge. If he then did better still, there would be another move, to maybe Barnet or Finchley. Mrs. Stuart's family had started in Whitechapel, and was now on the ladder. This most interesting of patients told me that she had two medical conditions that were almost unique to her, and that consultants in various hospitals had been unable to help her.

Mrs. Stuart was a new patient to the London, and so I had to take a full medical history. I asked her the standard questions, concerning whether she had ever suffered from cardiac problems, hepatitis, and so on. And then I enquired what her two unique medical conditions were.

"Well," she replied, beaming as though she was now going to divulge something that would truly amaze me, "You know that people have *seven* layers of skin......

I had not been taught that we had 'seven layers of skin', though I understood that there were ways in which the composition of skin could be described in that manner.

"Well," and she was beaming ever brightly, "I have just ONE!" With the final word she almost broke into a shout!

"Oh dear," I sympathized, "I am sorry to hear that. Does that mean that you have to be really careful that you don't injure yourself? How has it affected you?"

"It's the sun," she said, which probably beamed dimly in comparison to Mrs. Stuart at this moment. "It can shrivel me up. Just one layer, *one layer*, and so if the sun were to shine on me, I would just shrivel."

"How do you know that?" I enquired. "Have you been told that by a consultant? Has it ever happened, or started to happen?"

"No-one's told me," she replied. "I worked it out for myself. If I have only one layer of skin, and were to lay in the sun – *gone*! Just like that. Shrivelled."

"So how do you manage this condition?" I asked, quite intrigued by now.

"I keep myself well covered when the sun is out," she replied. "And my Izzy, he says he's embarrassed. I take his army greatcoat from the war to the beach when we go, and I wear it – and a broad brimmed hat. I like the beach, and Izzy does too, but I have to take precautions, you see. I've worked it all out."

"Might I enquire what the other medical condition is?" I ventured.

"It's my blood," she gushed. "It doesn't clot properly. As *you* know, normal blood clots like this....." and Mrs. Stuart proceeded to embark on a sort of hand-jive, with the right hand twisting over the left, then the two hands rolling round together, and coming to a sudden halt with the right hand placed horizontally over the left.

"But my blood clots like *this*...." and off went the hands again, rolling around together until suddenly the right hand, first finger fully extended, shot towards the ceiling, finishing in what resembled a Nazi salute.

"My blood clots like *that*," she proclaimed with barely concealed delight at my attentiveness. I could not resist temptation at this point, and asked her, "Could you show me that again please?", and started scribbling on her dental records.

Clearly this was a party trick that had been performed a hundred times before, and I could not help sparing a thought for poor 'Izzy'.

The animated hand-jive was taking place again, with the accompanying explanation, "Like *this*" and "As *you* know" and "Like *that*".

"Mrs. Stuart, this is quite an unusual condition, and I would like to ask you a kindness. Would you be willing to explain your blood clotting to a few of my colleagues, please? I know they would find it most interesting, and will probably not come across it again for a long time."

A word in the ear of a few of my fellow students, and soon a small crowd had gathered, as Mrs. Stuart's hands rolled and dived, passing over and over, and through each other, and finally ending in that salute!

"*Absolutely fascinating!*" said a senior dental tutor who had joined the assembled throng. "Please show me again," and so it continued for around fifteen minutes, after which everyone dispersed, whispering and smiling together. I wondered how Mrs. Stuart's blood clotting cabaret had started, and my best guess was that she had once seen a consultant who gesticulated greatly whilst explaining why a minor scratch or similar was slow to heal. I will never know of course, but it was one of those memorable and unforgettable moments during my clinical training back in the late 1960s.

By now, you may well be asking just where the patients we practiced on came from? They seemed to fall into three categories. Firstly, there were those who lived in the locality, and had always attended the London because it was their hospital, they wanted to support the students, and it would never enter their thinking to go anywhere else. These people were our core patients, and we loved them. They knew the area and its history, they knew all the stall holders, they knew each other – and they usually knew the Kray brothers!

The second category was people who travelled in from a modest distance because the treatment was free. They knew we were students who were learning and practicing, but they also knew that there were always staff tutors watching, and that we were expected to work to a high standard, even though it would mean longer appointments. Some treatments, such as bridges, were not so often carried out in general dental practice in those days, but at the hospital we rather enjoyed carrying out more advanced procedures – and there was no charge to the patient.

The third category of people treated by students was those whose dental treatment was deemed to be too advanced or complicated to be undertaken by their dental practitioner. And so the dentist would refer them to a consultant at the London, who would sometimes take a look at them and say, "It's not *that* complicated – give them to a student." People who had impacted wisdom teeth, or recurring gum disease, or dentures that they could not get on with often arrived at the London, relieved that someone of stature was going to look after them – and were given to a student! They would be reassured that all treatment would be done under close supervision, and a senior registrar or consultant would take over if the procedure did indeed become rather complicated.

By this time Sheila and I were seeing each other almost daily. She had moved from her Hall of Residence into a flat, with three other physiotherapists. To many of my fellow dental students, she was known as 'Green Stamps'. "So how are you getting on with Green Stamps?" and "What are you and Green Stamps doing at the weekend?" were questions certain of my colleagues would ask. Green Stamps? – a company had started a scheme called 'Green Shield Stamps', and I was hooked on it. Many shops, but by no means all, offered Green Shield stamps with purchases, and I had a book in which I collected the stamps. When the book was full I could exchange it for goods, such as an iron, or an electric toaster – for free! Sheila, too, started looking for the Green Shield symbol in shop windows and doorways, and having bought the goods and obtained the stamps, passed them on to me. This, I told myself, was true love indeed, but many of my dental colleagues simply referred to Sheila as 'Green Stamps'.

My government grant was modest, and I had to be careful with regard to expenditure. Another financial factor was that dental students did not have a summer break of two or three months, as did most students at that time, and so could not supplement their grant by working for the summer. Our courting, therefore, took the form of inexpensive activities, such as walking down to the docks at Wapping. It was an interesting part of the city, and had not changed much since Victorian times, and we would wander hand-in-hand through streets that still showed the bomb damage from the Second World War, and sit on some wooden steps that led down to the water itself, on a wharf, and gaze out across the Thames. Various boats carrying a variety of freight and cargo would sail slowly by as we sat and discussed everything and nothing, as lovers do. I remember one evening when I had used some of my meagre grant to buy Sheila a peach, and produced it as a treat for her to enjoy as we sat and watched the oily water drift by. Was it me, or was it Sheila? It does not matter, but one of us dropped the peach, and we sat there and watched helplessly as the peach, almost in slow motion, bounced from step to step...... plop... plop... plop...and eventually, splash! We both felt so sad about that peach – the sacrificial giving and the anticipated enjoyment. These days I buy peaches in multiples of four, but it was all so different as a student in the East End of London in those days. And there was the occasional excursion to the local Indian restaurant, and sometimes the Chinese restaurant, though these were rare treats.

I wanted Sheila to meet my parents, and for them to meet her, and so we made the journey back to Norfolk, where everyone was on their best behavior, and no doubt some wondered whether wedding bells were in the offing. Certainly not on our grants, and at this time we were still looking at a further two years study, not realizing that I would have to do an additional year, making it three. Then Sheila's parents came up to London, staying in a rather posh hotel right in the centre of the city. Her father had a builder's merchants business just outside Exeter, though neither of us was quite sure what that involved. I thought bricks, and Sheila was fairly certain that coal was involved. We enjoyed dinner together one evening, and I thought that Sheila's mother's West Country accent was rather attractive, and they might well have thought that by contrast, people from Norfolk were complete yokels! But the "Oi in't got an accint" was starting to flatten out.

Now that I was a believer – in fact, I was totally convinced, and have been ever since, which seems to be verging on the unreasonable to some people! – there was nothing to stop us romancing, being a couple, and looking towards a possible future together. It was some time before either of us brought the subject up, and when we did so, it was in a somewhat vague way, and we spoke in generalities at that time. As I stated earlier, I have always been of mediocre academic ability, and regularly studied from 7 p.m. to around 2 a.m. and that after a very full 9 to 5 day in the clinics, laboratories and lecture theatres. But there was always time to see Sheila, and most days we would have time at least for a coffee and a catch up on the day's news.

We found a small church along a road called Stepney Way, and would attend there together on Sunday evenings. The minister was helpful to me in those early days as a Christian, as were a number of the medical students and a dental student, two years below me, called Richard. One couple in the church, of late middle age and with a strong Scottish accent, came over to us on our first visit, and insisted that we called round for supper one evening during the week. The address was 4 Lindley Street, as I heard it, and their surname was Warthog, as I heard it. An evening was agreed, and we found Lindley Street, and we found number 4, but it was empty, and still showing the scars of bomb damage. Were they 'down and outs' showing kindness to two poor students? We trudged back to Sheila's flat, had a sandwich or two, and I returned to my studies. The following Sunday we were assailed with "Wee deed ye naw cawm to our hoose?" and after some animated conversation found that they in fact lived at number 4 *Leslie* Street. Even to this day I have difficulty understanding anyone with an accent – Scottish, Irish, Asian, any, to my embarrassment at times – and yet there was more to come. We were again invited to supper with these dear people, later that week, but the following evening, I wrote them a letter apologizing for my mistake, and put it through their letter box. When we arrived later in the week for supper with them, I was assailed again. They were not the 'Mr. and Mrs. Warthog' I had addressed my apologetic letter to, but 'Mr. and Mrs. *Wardhaugh*'. Fortunately they were very gracious people, and we became firm friends, and called round for coffee after church nearly every Sunday evening for the rest of our time there.

I was not knowledgeable about this new Person who had changed my entire life, so it seemed, by actually changing *me*. I felt that getting to know more about the God of the Bible was a priority, and so I put 15 minutes aside each day for reading the Scriptures. I loved reading the Bible, and so often it seemed almost alive with information that I 'devoured' it in the way a ravenous man attacks steak and chips. I also wanted to get to know the Person himself, and spent a further 15 minutes in prayer each day. In fact, midnight to half-midnight became an almost sacred time, and was very special. Much of prayer time was just enjoying God's presence, and involved thanking him for being so good to me, and worship. These things often seem incomprehensible to the unbeliever, and had done to me – but now it was as if a veil had been covering my understanding, and that it had at last been lifted. And occasionally I would ask things in prayer, and sometimes get a negative response, but both Sheila and I can remember well a time when we prayed together about how I could make ends meet on such a modest grant. I had stopped having lunch each day, as I just did not have the money. My grant had not increased much from my first year, but I was in London many more weeks a year, and it had to stretch further. We went to church that Sunday evening, and the minister said at the start of his sermon, "I feel I should speak about money this evening....." and unknowingly answered all the questions Sheila and I had asked in prayer. It was what the sceptic calls a coincidence, but there are just far too many of them for the Christian to believe that – and more fool the sceptic for thinking so.

Sheila had a Jewish landlord, and he and his family ran a small corner shop a stone's throw from the hospital. I quite often went in there, which could be an interesting experience. There were coins in those days called half-crowns (equivalent to twelve and a half pence today) and other coins called florins (ten pence today). Such amounts of money went a lot further in those days, of course. If I or anyone paid with one of these coins, they would immediately examine the date. I forget the exact details, but a half-crown dated earlier than say, 1920, would contain silver worth, say twenty pence, and could be sold on for such. And those prior to say, 1938, could also be sold for a premium – and were. But that couple had hearts of gold (not silver) and when they found that I was Sheila's boyfriend, and was a student, absolutely *insisted* that I have lunch in their home every Tuesday. And so I did, though they were always – *always* – too busy to join me. And lunch was always three courses, and the main course was always steak, served by their au pair girl. There was little I could do to show my gratitude, though there were occasions when I would join my host on his trips to clubs across the East End of London, where he had cigarette machines. I guarded the crates of cigarettes while he refilled the machines, because he said he knew what would happen to 'the fags' if he turned his back.

Sheila and I had been an item for over a year, and we realized that we wanted to marry. I said nothing directly to Sheila about it, nor she to me, but whilst we were staying in Exeter with her parents for a weekend, looked for an opportunity to ask her father's consent. Finding the moment seemed impossible, but when he announced that he was going to drive to Taunton to collect his son from boarding school, I asked if I could go with him. And then I lost my nerve, as almost pure adrenaline seemed to flow through my veins. With a relatively short distance to go, I suddenly blurted out, "How would you feel about me marrying your daughter?" and he immediately braked sharply, bringing his BMW down to what seemed like a crawl. He was not a man of many words, and was obviously carefully weighing up his response. When he did, it was absolutely textbook; "What are your prospects?" he asked. My prospects? Well, I hoped to eventually pass my exams and qualify as a dentist, and then I simply wanted to go into general practice, and treat ordinary people like myself, and settle down and have a family, and grow old and enjoy my grandchildren. He was silent for a minute or two, and the suspense was almost too much for me, until he said that he and his wife had assumed that Sheila and I might want to marry, that we appeared well-suited, and they would give us their blessing. I explained that I had not yet asked Sheila, of course, but would look for an opportunity in the near future.

The 'near future' was in fact, Valentine's Day, and we were again at a 'hop' and in the same hall where I had first set eyes on Sheila. We were taking a break from dancing and had gone to the bar in the balcony overlooking the dance floor, when I said I had a question for her. She was unsuspecting, as it happened, and when I asked her she almost fainted. In fact, she felt so weak that she asked if she could go to my room and lay down for a while, and I helped support her along the corridors, as the dance hall was in the students hostel where I lived.

The next day we set out to buy a ring, and Sheila knew exactly what she wanted – a sapphire ring. I would have guessed that a sapphire was blue, but did not really know about such things. We came to a shop in Hatton Garden where there was 'just what she wanted', and I slipped it on her finger and we floated back to Whitechapel, where having blown several months grant on the ring, I was uncharacteristically extravagant again and took her to dinner to a restaurant called the Poor Millionaire. We talked a lot about getting married, and thought we would have two children, a boy and a girl just like my parents, and be the ideal family. I was on course for qualifying at the end of 1967, and so maybe in the spring of 1968.......

And then I failed a vital exam in the summer of 1967, which was so strange in view of the work I had put in. I was told I could not take finals that December, and would be retaking my 'denture exam' at that time, and could not in fact take my finals until the following summer. That December, on the day of my exam, I developed 'flu and felt dreadful. I turned up anyway, because I needed to pass and wanted to get married – but failed dismally. I had to appear before the dean, who said maybe I should give up, and that if I failed again I would have to leave the dental school. The county authorities who gave me my grant said they would have to review the situation, but also decided to give me one more chance. Sheila came round every evening, and went through old exam papers, asking me question after question in order that I might, if possible, know even more about dentures than the examiners themselves. And that summer I passed the exam with ease, and in the December took my finals, where I was examined on everything I had ever been taught at the hospital, from the anteater's lack of teeth to the latest advance in gum surgery and bridge materials, and carried out fillings whilst observed by stern looking men in white coats.

And I passed! It seemed unbelievable to me, and indeed for months I would have dreams that I was sitting my finals and that my mind was blank. I would wake up believing that I had failed, and only as I consciously thought back to the moment of seeing my name on the college notice board as a 'pass', would I feel that relief again.

"Lawrence has passed?" said one of the tutors who had never really liked me, and especially so following my conversion after which my consumption of alcohol diminished rather significantly; the tutor, in fact, who had thrown out the debagging challenge that very first year at the annual Dental Dinner. "Lawrence has passed? That is like letting a monkey loose with a pistol," he added to the hoots of everyone present in the Sammie that evening. But I was not there to hear it, though there were those who made sure I did – I was off to the Veeraswamy Restaurant in Swallow Street, which in those days was in the Victorian style of the Raj, and where waiters in turbans saluted, and bowed, and made me feel as if I really had qualified at last as a professional.

And then life took some interesting turns!

CHAPTER 7

Kissing the Bride, Kissing the Daisies, and the Dog Tooth!

My parents had been so excited when I had first decided to be a dentist, and had shown great interest in my course and life in London. I do not think that anyone – *anyone* – in our family had ever been to a university before. Indeed, it was a tiny minority of those leaving school in those days that actually went on to higher education, although it has become almost expected of so many young people today.

Having learnt that I had qualified at last, I caught the train back to North Walsham and spent that Christmas with my parents. After that, I had to pick up my car. My car? Yes, I had briefly had a car, when, on my twenty-first birthday my parents announced that they had been paying into a savings scheme for me, and it was now complete. They presented me with a cheque for £320, which was quite a useful sum of money at that time. I wanted a car, like the rich boys at university, and soon found a 1956 Hillman Minx that (together with tax and insurance) came into my price range. I had swanned around London in it for a few months, taking Sheila out in style, and yet struggling to actually run it. And then in the late spring of 1966 I was driving to Southend for a day on the beach, when all the traffic came to a halt – except me. I hit the car in front quite badly, and Sheila was taken to hospital with a cut leg. The police did not charge me, and my Uncle Sidney, who had a car repair business in Hertfordshire and was always so kind to me, put it back together. However, the insurance company wanted a shed-full of money if I was to go back on the road – and so that was the end of my University driving days. But at Christmas 1968 I retrieved it from my uncle and insured it again. I was back on the road and heading south.

The road from North Walsham wound its way to Norwich, and continued to wind and meander south towards London, with some towns and villages being legendary bottlenecks. Skirting London and heading southwest on the A30 took me through Hampshire, Wiltshire and down into Dorset. The rolling chalk hills told me that Shaftesbury was not so far, and at last I arrived in that most delightful of towns. Reg, the dentist whose practice it was, had arranged for me to stay on a farm just outside the town; in fact, he had stayed there himself when he had first arrived three years previously as an associate of the previous practice owner, before buying the practice.

The arrangement was that I would have a room, and break-fast and an evening meal would be included. Mrs. Parrott, the farmer's wife, would do my washing and ironing. I soon settled in, and slowly became accustomed to the aroma of what was politely called 'cow muck', the cows themselves sometimes trumpeting through the night, and Mr. Parrott snoring as he slept at various times of the day on the tatty sofa by the log burner, straw protruding from his jacket pockets and hair.

After over five years of studying in an environment of brick, concrete, glass, and Tarmac; of coping with the jostling, rushing, and pushing, and people, people, people..... being kept awake by the trumpeting of a cow or the hoot of an owl was music to my ears, and the heavy aroma of 'cow muck' was amazingly refreshing.

The Parrotts were of late middle age, kindly country folk with round fresh faces, and portly frames clad in soiled bestrawed clothing that had seen far better days. The farm-house became my home for four months, while I learnt how to fill in NHS forms and to adapt my student, city hospital dentistry to that of a rural practice. The needles were not of the disposable type that we had used in dental school, but re-usable and needing to be sterilised between patients. They were suspended in an antiseptic solution in something resembling a spaghetti jar, which was on a cabinet directly in front of the patient. However, disposable needles were starting to find their way into general practice, and were to make a big difference to the experience of patients attending for fillings and extractions. I could remember only too well the extreme discomfort of having the roof of my mouth numbed at around the age of ten, in order to have my upper molars extracted. It had been horrendous. But re-using the older non-disposable needles was much more economic than using the newer ones and throwing them away, and this factor needed to be taken into consideration by dentists trying to maintain the viability of their NHS practices.

The economics of running a Health Service dental practice was one of the hard facts of life that I had to get used to, especially where laboratory work was involved. This could be a major expense, and dentists were ever looking for the cheapest laboratory. The Shaftesbury practice had its own lab in a small room at the rear of the building, and Harry would sit with his wax and Bunsen burner, setting up trial dentures and later processing them. He had once been a dentist - before one had to train or qualify. "Just used to pull 'em art," said the London-born mechanic. "Me and me mate got so drunk one night, that when 'e said 'e 'ad the longest roots in London, I took 'im back to my place and pulled 'em *all* art!" He grinned broadly. "''is missus came round cursin' me the next day, demanding free teeth for 'er Fred.... I 'ad to do 'em really. Matter of honour." And then the government passed the Dentists Act in 1921 and anyone wanting to practise dentistry had to pay £5 and register. Harry did not think it was worth £5 to be a dentist, so he carried on without paying it, and was the first one prosecuted for doing so. He paid a £5 fine at Bow Street Magistrates

Court and changed career, from untrained dentist to untrained dental technician. By the time he retired to Shaftesbury, he was rather good at it, and promptly came out of retirement in order to supplement his pension. He too had encountered Christ on his own Damascus Road, and was now a teetotal, committed member of the local Baptist church, and sometimes preached around the area.

Back at the London we had been working in a world isolated from economic reality, but now in practice there were bills to pay as well as patients to treat. We wanted to do our best, but we also needed to stay viable. The idealist went bankrupt and the outright profiteer carried out poor treatment, and most of us were trying to steer a course avoiding bankruptcy whilst maintaining good treatment standards.

There was another dentist in the area who could have been seen as a competitor, and a local dental committee had to decide periodically whether he was still fit to practise. The fact that he had lost an eye in a brawl in a local bar rendered him handicapped when the need for 3D vision was required (cavity depth, for example). He had set up his practice many years previously when there were few regulations governing the practice of dentistry, and the dental chair in his dining room was next to the sideboard, where the compartments in the cutlery drawer were for knives, forks, spoons, mirrors, probes, and tweezers. Forceps were in the next drawer, with serviettes and corkscrews. Local dentists always suggested the committee 'keep him on a little longer,' and one of them explained to me that we didn't want 'anybody sensible working there.'

My first year in practice was my worst, as I felt so inadequate. Too often I would whisper to my nurse, "What do I do?" and sometimes she knew and sometimes she didn't. But after around a year there, I started to feel at ease in the surgery, and began carrying out more sophisticated treatments. "When you win the lottery, come and ask me about bridges," I would say to people with a missing tooth, and they would realise firstly, that there was an alternative to a denture, and secondly, that it would be expensive. Some came back and asked, and some proceeded with treatment. "Why are you doing so many bridges?" asked Reg, surprised that people would ask *me* to carry out such treatment.

I liked the work and I loved the patients. Also, *holey* teeth had become *holy* teeth, and this had practical implications. It sounds horribly pious, but teeth are part of this wonderful creation – God made them! And teeth are simply a part of a person, and that person is made in the image of God – people are important. So I treated *people*, not teeth, and everything I did to the teeth and gums was within the context of God's creation.

I'm not sure I had ever heard of Shaftesbury before the position at the practice came to my attention. It was all part of what seemed to be a wonderful adventure. Enjoying the presence of God was adding a whole new dimension to life, and was having practical implications. When my finals were approaching, I realized that before long I would need to find somewhere to work, and Sheila and I had talked about this. Sheila's father owned property, and one house had three dental surgeries, two of which were occupied and one vacant. It seemed an obvious move to plan to go to Exeter and use that surgery. And then, with the time getting close, there were problems. Sheila's father explained that he was going to be in dispute with the dentists who worked there with regard to the rent they paid, and did not want me involved in it. Suddenly I had nowhere to work, and I was not sure how to find a position in general practice.

It was at this point that one of my Christian friends told me that the Lord has a plan for each of our lives, and often this means following what looks like the normal course, and to accept that he will block it if it is not his will. Certainly my 'normal course' seemed well and truly blocked. My friend then took me to an incident in the life of the apostle Paul, where on one of his missionary journeys the normal course would have been to go to Bithynia, but it was blocked. The Lord then showed him that he should instead go to Macedonia. My friend showed me the passage in Acts 16, and suggested I ask the Lord what his direction was for me at this time. Within a few days a letter arrived from a man who had been part of a team that Sheila and I had joined during the summer, working with a mission to children on Sheringham beach in Norfolk. The man said that he had just heard of a Christian dentist in Shaftesbury who had too much work and was looking for help, and gave me his name and telephone number. It was just another of that string of 'coincidences' that happen to Christians – in other words, God! I had telephoned the practice, went to meet the dentist, and having passed my finals, now found myself working there.

During my first few months in Shaftesbury, I returned to London on three occasions. Firstly there was the degree ceremony which was to take place at the Royal Albert Hall, and where the Queen Mother, the Chancellor of the University, would present me with my degree. Well, along with a few thousand others, and maybe she would not hand it to me in person. I was given two guest tickets, and I assumed that Sheila and my parents would want to be there, so what should I do? But my parents lived some distance away, and probably did not realize the significance of the ceremony. So Sheila came with me, and watched as I strode across the platform, pausing to give a stiff little bow towards Her Majesty, before exiting stage left where my degree was thrust into my hand by a minion.

The second excursion was to take another examination. My degree was awarded by the University, but some of the older dentists did not have a degree, but a qualification of equivalent value awarded by the Royal College of Surgeons of England. This was a 'licence' to practice dentistry, and I felt that to have this, in addition to my degree, might just possibly be useful at some time in the future. The attraction was that if I applied within twelve months of obtaining my degree, I could take just the finals of the LDS (Licence in Dental Surgery) and not the three years of exams leading up to it (though I would be charged for those other exams). So I drove up to London and sat the finals of the LDS exam.

It was a month or two later when, for the third time, I again drove to the big city, this time to find out whether or not I had passed. It was not so important for me, but for many it was their last chance having failed the degree, perhaps more than once already. The manner of informing us, and there were around forty assembled there, must have been unique, for we had to gather in a hallway at the foot of a rather stately staircase. Halfway up the staircase was a door, and there was a second door at the top of the staircase. We waited. Eventually the door halfway up the staircase opened, and a rather lean, poker-faced man, resembling to my mind an undertaker, emerged and stared dispassionately at us. Silence! He produced a sheet of paper and read from it in a monotone.

"Abednego Josiah Charles Awolowe." A tall African walked forward and slowly ascended the staircase until he reached the undertaker.

"Passed," said the dispassionate one, and with visible relief on his face Mr. Awolowe continued up the staircase and stood by the door at the top.

"Benjamin Arthur McCarter Brown," and Mr. McCarter Brown stepped forward and slowly ascended to the poker-faced man.

"Failed," hissed the miserable man of death, and there was a tangible feeling of grief for the poor man who now had to turn round and walk back down to the rest of us – and out through the entrance door. Slowly and alphabetically, the silent assembly at the foot of the stairs shrank in number.

"Barrie Richard Lawrence," droned the undertaker, and my heart started to pound as I ascended, step by step, to stand just below him, to hear...

"Passed."

With great relief I mounted the remaining steps to join the other successful candidates standing by the top door. Around 30% had been sent back down, and there was a great hush as the door at the top opened and another sober gentleman beckoned us in, and directed us to form a line along the wall at the back of the room.

In front of us were heavy oak desks, with a number of chairs, and while we were all taking in the scene, a door to our right opened and a number of berobed, very elderly gentlemen entered, with three of them carrying items of regalia which I thought might have included an orb, a mace and a sceptre, though my knowledge of such matters is virtually non-existent. But they looked very stately and important as they sat down whilst another man of dignity read out our names and stated that we were now being welcomed into the Royal College of Surgeons of England. The berobed gentlemen then arose, and their chief asked us to repeat after him the Hippocratic Oath. We followed the man, sentence by sentence, and I cannot remember a word of it, but the essence of the oath is that the practitioner swears that he will always put the patient's interests first and treat them to the very best of his or her ability, regardless of payment, ethnicity, religion, etc. etc. And so we swore.

And then these great ones, and of such dignity, broke out in smiles, and fairly chuckling, said "Well done chaps" and came out from behind their desks and shook hands with each of us and, still chortling and chuckling, vanished through another door and were gone. At this we turned back to the door by which we had entered and descended the staircase to the hall, and left.

I never really used that qualification, having no desire to advance in terms of further academic studies or engage in much hospital work. However, there was a distinct advantage, which only became apparent with the passing of time. I had the letters BDS (Bachelor of Dental Surgery) after my name, like most of my dental colleagues, but was now entitled to also have LDS RCS (England) for Licence in Dental Surgery, Royal College of Surgeons, or LDS RCSE – and I chose the latter. The advantage that came from this was that some prospective patients apparently count the letters after a professional's name, and whereas most of my colleagues had three, I now had ten. I was no better qualified, and yet was told by one beaming lady that I had "more letters after your name than any other dentist in the Yellow Pages." The result was that I had new patients, who did not know me from Adam, travelling significant distances to see 'the man with all the letters.'

* * * * * * * * * *

But there was a wedding being planned, and many weekends I would drive down to Exeter in my rotting Hillman Minx and spend time with Sheila and her family. The wedding was to be there on 24th May at the Methodist Church in the centre of town. After the wedding service, we would walk out of the church and find ourselves on a bus-stop, but there would be a Rolls Royce waiting to take us to the hotel where the reception would take place. We would have the photographs taken in the gardens there, and proceed into the hotel and form a line with parents to shake the hands of the guests, and so on and so forth. Mr. Heywood (my future father-in-law) was always gracious and kind and helpful, and also extremely generous with regard to the expense of the wedding, paying for hire of the morning suits we would be wearing, as well as the reception.

Sheila and I would go for walks, or even on occasions cycle down to the coast, where we would wander along beaches hand in hand, and talk about our future together. Time seemed to pass rather slowly in those days, and the few months running up to the wedding seemed like an age, but the day eventually arrived. Richard, a fellow Christian dental student who had been with me in the Students Hostel, was my best man. Sheila looked even more beautiful, the bridesmaids had forgotten their hats but looked cute, we got our responses right, and I was told I could kiss the bride. We travelled to the reception in a Rolls Royce and not on a double-decker bus, and I somehow got through my speech. I cannot remember what I said, though I can still remember some of the gracious content of that of my new father-in-law.

We ran through a storm of confetti to our car (I had changed the Hillman for a Ford Anglia Estate), and drove to Glastonbury for our first night, and then proceeded to Wales for our honeymoon. For two weeks we walked beaches, had romantic meals, strolled up Snowdon barely a few yards in front of Prince Charles and Lord Snowdon (it was just prior to the former's Investiture as Prince of Wales – we wondered why there were so many helicopters in the area). We wished our timing had been better as we might have met them. We then returned to Shaftesbury, where we rented a small bungalow. We had ordered some new furniture, but there was a strike at the factory, and so we borrowed two deck chairs, an orange box, and a picnic table. After supper in the kitchen, we would pick up our deck chairs, take them through to the sitting room and spend the rest of the evening there. One day the furniture finally arrived – but we had good memories of those early days.

* * * * * * * * * *

The people in Shaftesbury were warm and friendly, and we enjoyed our years there. Our first two daughters were born in the town, and in addition to finding a few decent restaurants, a squash club and making some good friends, I started to preach in local churches and organize tent crusades for the evangelist Don Double, with whom I had become friendly.

And as always, where there are people there are humorous incidents. Or is it just the way some of us look at life?

A man in his thirties, wearing a long dark coat and with intense staring eyes had walked into the surgery. I gave him a smile, and said "Do take your coat off, and come and sit down." However, he kept his coat on, and with his eyes fixed on the chair proceeded to slowly walk round it, twice clockwise, pausing, and then going once more round it in the other direction. It was as if he was performing some religious rite, and Sarah, my nurse, and I remained motionless and silently observed. He then climbed onto the footrest, and proceeded to kneel on the seat facing over the back of the headrest.

"Would you prefer to turn round and sit the other way?" I enquired, but he had made up his mind, and whilst continuing to kneel backwards on the chair, he fumbled in his coat pocket and extracted what I assumed was, maybe a list of medication that I would need to know about. But it was nothing of the sort, and when I approached he showed me a photograph of a group of people, and explained "That's Uncle Bert, and this one is Uncle George."

"How interesting," I said, and was asking myself how we proceeded from there, when he volunteered, "It's the *dog* tooth."

"Oh, I see. It's the dog tooth," I said, expressing gratitude for the information, and enquired, "Which dog tooth is that?"

"The *dog* tooth," he continued, "This one," and he rested his finger on his upper left canine. "Want it out," he continued, and I could see that it was extensively decayed, and when I rested my finger on the tooth it was obviously painful, indicating an abscess.

"You have an abscess and need antibiotic tablets to get rid of the infection before I take it out," I explained. "No," he replied, "Want it out," and I somehow felt he was not going to get out of my chair until his tooth had been extracted.

"Perhaps you would like to sit round, and I can inject it for you," I said.

"No. Do it here," he said, staring through the rear surgery wall in front of him.

I considered the situation, and felt that not much was going to change unless I fitted in with the patient's wishes, and so I loaded my syringe with anaesthetic and walked round to the back of the chair where I found he had opened his mouth. I gave the two injections necessary for the extraction of the tooth, and offered him a rinse, but he silently shook his head. Around five minutes later I went to the back of the chair again, and used my forceps to remove the tooth. This time he climbed out of the chair and stood to have a rinse, and then said "Thank you dentist" before walking out of the surgery and signing the appropriate NHS forms at reception.

He would occasionally return with one problem or another, seemed to regard me as his friend, usually showed me family photographs, and always sat in the chair in the conventional manner at subsequent visits.

Mr. Pickles was a different case altogether. A rep for a large company and a regular patient attending every six months for a check-up, he would book an appointment early in the day. He always wore a suit on his portly frame, shook hands with me on entering the surgery and exchanged the usual pleasantries. The day arrived when Mr. Pickles needed his first filling. As I slowly injected the gum beside the tooth I could see beads of perspiration gathering on his brow. As I withdrew the needle Mr. Pickles contorted his face and roared "Arrrgggh-hhhh!," pushed me out of the way, flung open the door and tore out of the surgery. It was what I imagined a horror movie to be like, and I stood rooted to the spot, as did Sarah on the far side of the surgery.

I left the surgery through the open door and found that the front door to the practice at the end of the hallway was also open. Outside there was a heavy dew, and clear tracks round the side of the building in the grass, and I followed them over the lawn to the rear of the practice garden, where Mr. Pickles was lying face down in the long, soaking wet grass – motionless. I bent down and took his wrist to check for a pulse, only to find him turn his head and say, "It's OK old boy. I'm just kissing the daisies!"

"Oh, I see," was all I could say. Mr. Pickles continued, "I'll be back soon." And so I went back to the surgery, and sure enough within five or so minutes Mr. Pickles re-entered, his grey suit almost dripping at the front. He returned to the chair, saying "Sorry about that", and I continued to carry out the filling as if nothing had happened. Curiously, Mr. Pickles usually clambered out of the chair after an injection, and made a one-man stampede for the door, down the hall and out into the garden to 'kiss the daisies'. So when Mr. Pickles was booked in for a procedure requiring an injection, we always allowed additional 'daisy-kissing time'.

And then there was Neville – the same Neville who had lost his nerve and hidden in the woodyard. You will remember that Neville was a new patient, and appeared to have lost his nerve, and legged it. I left the story with Neville hiding behind timber in a woodyard a few hundred yards from the surgery, while I paced up and down, unable to find him and wondering what I should do next.

My decision was to continue on to the hotel where Neville worked, and as the manager there had brought him round to the practice, I would explain to him what had happened. The man seemed to understand absolutely, as he had apparently been taking Neville to the town doctor a few weeks previously when he had raced off after a bus pulling away from the kerb, leapt on, and travelled the twenty or so miles to Salisbury, from whence he had to be retrieved. Neville did not have an affinity towards health professionals.

While the manager and I were conversing, his telephone rang. It was my surgery to say that Neville had returned and was sitting in the chair as if nothing had happened, and so I returned to the practice.

I resisted the temptation to greet the man with "Nice day for hiding in a woodyard", and quietly washed my hands and asked Neville how I could help him. He simply closed his eyes and opened his mouth to reveal pink gums and black circles. Every tooth had rotted off at gum level leaving a black circle of root on the surface. As many teeth have two or three roots, there were probably around forty roots present. I asked him if he was in pain, and he shook his head. Maybe he would like me to make him a set of dentures with which to smile and eat his food – and he slowly nodded. I explained that this would require the removal of the roots that were present, and Neville gave no response. If he would like me to proceed....... and I outlined the number and duration of appointments, and what I would be doing at each. I explained that I would tell him at each visit what I would be doing, and also what I would be doing at the following visit. Amazingly, Neville never missed an appointment, was always on time, and quietly sat in the chair and had every root extracted, impressions taken for dentures and the various stages leading up to the day when I fitted them. I handed him a mirror, and the previously shrunken, wrinkled cheeks and sad face now beamed with a broad grin like a Cheshire cat!

"You may well need me to adjust your new teeth," I explained, and told him to return if he had any pain from them. We shook hands, and after smiling his way to reception to sign the relevant NHS forms, Neville grinned his way down the hallway and strode off in the direction of the hotel.

A happy ending? So it seemed, but life takes some strange turns, and around a week later, one of the hotel reception staff came to the practice bearing a large envelope, and handing it to me said, "Neville says 'Can you do something?'"

I opened the envelope and peered in to find, perhaps around fifty fragments of pink and white plastic. Neville's dentures were beyond repair. I enquired how his teeth had come to be in so many tiny fragments, and the story the girl told me ensured that I would never again take my wife to dine at that hotel.

Neville had been employed by the hotel as a dish-washer, as this was before the days of mechanical ones. Around the same time, the hotel had taken on a new vegetable chef, who was a rough, thuggish man (eventually to be dismissed for threatening the manager with a broken beer mug, whilst drunk). The vegetable chef would taunt the rather diminutive and timid dish-washer with insults, until the latter responded with something similar. At this point the vegetable chef would swear at Neville, reach into his mouth and, extracting his upper and lower dentures, hurl them across the hotel kitchen at the dish-washer who, with the rest of the kitchen staff, would dive for cover. The chef would then stride across the room, pick up his teeth and put them back in his mouth. As the staff were in fear of the man, no-one intervened or reported him and his reign of terror in the kitchen continued until Neville had a great idea, leading him to attend the surgery, lose his nerve, regain it and persevere with visits until he too had a set of false teeth.

Back in the hotel kitchen, and grinning at the rest of the staff, Neville waited for the inevitable taunts, "You 'orrible little man, you" and "Where *did* you get those teeth?" and so on. "'orrible man yourself," he responded, and stuck his tongue out. As the vegetable chef pulled out his dentures, the kitchen staff ducked behind cabinets. He flung his teeth across the kitchen, as Neville swerved to his left, removed his own teeth and threw them with all his might at the chef. The big bully of a man stamped down with his foot – CRUNCH! – and then again – CRUNCH! – and quickly strode across the kitchen to regain his own teeth, leaving around fifty small pieces of pink and white plastic for the tearful Neville to collect, and send to me in an envelope.

I told the girl to suggest to Neville that he return to the surgery so that I could make him a new set of false teeth – but I never saw him again after that incident. Maybe he moved on to pastures new. Shortly after that the vegetable chef was sacked, and I found a different hotel in a different town where Sheila and I could enjoy dinner out from time to time.

* * * * * * * * *

These were the days when dentists in general practice still used gas and oxygen, especially for extracting children's teeth, and when requested by adults too. I did not really enjoy them - and nor did the patients! One stage in the onset of anaesthesia is the 'excitability stage', and we were never sure what would happen at that point. My most memorable recollection of this stage was when a large gypsy attended to have a tooth extracted, and requested "Gas!" Looking back, it was rather barbaric in that we would sit the patient in our cast iron upright dental chair, and then place one heavy duty strap over their knees to keep their legs and feet down, and another round their chest to prevent them leaving the chair forwards. However, our gypsy patient started rocking backwards and forwards, and then the cast iron chair started rocking with him. I was standing behind the patient, holding the mask over his face and trying to hang onto him as the chair rocked backwards and forwards, advancing each time by a few inches across the surgery towards Reg, who was trying to extract the tooth whilst walking backwards to prevent being assaulted by the chair bearing down on him. Somehow, we all survived the experience, but this was one reason that caused me to consider alternative ways that would be less traumatic for both patient and dentist.

On a course in Exeter on the subject of general anaesthetics, a doctor in general practice told me that he gave 'gas' for his local dentist. On one occasion the patient was sitting in the chair, the doctor had the mask in place, and after a couple of minutes or so, the patient's eyes rolled up, and then his eyelids closed. He was breathing regularly, and the doctor waited a further minute or so before looking across at the dentist, nodding towards the forceps, and saying "OK?"

"I'm fine thanks!" said the patient with his eyes still closed, to the surprise of both doctor and dentist. Those were strange days!

For surgery in hospitals, an intravenous anaesthetic was used, and having met a new young doctor in the town, I paid him a visit and enquired whether it was feasible to use this in general dental practice. He seemed enthusiastic about joining me for some intravenous sessions, and we decided to select appropriate patients where extractions were to be carried out. The patients were those too nervous for a local anaesthetic (injection) and probably too nervous for gas, and who said that an intravenous anaesthetic was what they wanted. It was all new to me, and the young doctor and I read what we could find on the subject, and prepared for our first session.

Colin, the enthusiastic young doctor, would inject a barbiturate into a vein in the patient's arm, and the effect would be immediate. I would go straight in with the forceps, and then we would try and bring them round. That took time, and even when they came round, they were very disorientated for some time. Our method of overcoming this would be deemed foolhardy and unprofessional today, but we would ask the patient to have a relative bring a car to the front gate, or they sometimes booked a taxi. Once the patient showed signs of recovery, Colin would take their ankles while I picked them up by their armpits, and with the nurse opening the doors ahead of us, we would run down the front path to the gate with the patient slung between us, and lay them out on the back seat of the vehicle, giving the driver instructions to 'drive carefully'.

Colin and I had several such sessions, but were quite understandably asked to end them by the practice owner as an audience would start assembling on the pavement opposite the practice when it became known that such a session was about to take place. They did not applaud or cheer, but stood and grinned and whispered to one another. Many years later when I had my own practice back in Norfolk, I went on courses at various London hospitals and learnt how to undertake such procedures properly, and carried out literally hundreds of intravenous anaesthetics and sedations on patients.

* * * * * * * * * *

Towards the end of my first year in Shaftesbury Sheila and I bought our first property. It was a small three-bedroomed bungalow on a new estate ten minutes walk from the practice. We did our first DIY decorating with emulsion and wallpaper, including one room in which we placed a cot, as our first baby would be born just two months later. The two of us were to become three, and life would never be quite the same again. Sarah was born on 28th February the following year, and I was present at the birth. I could not believe how beautiful she was, and felt like dancing for joy round the delivery room. Those days were very special, and a little under two years later she was joined by Rachel. They were so beautiful (and still are) and such a delight.

* * * * * * * * * *

When I first arrived in Shaftesbury I had visited two or three of the town's churches, and sat through the services. However, I had heard about a rather novel church that met a little over forty miles away, just south of Chard. Novel, in that it was so much like the church I read about in my New Testament. I was fascinated, and having driven over there and met some of the people, I decided to travel there as often as possible. Why drive so far? Let me tell you a few things about that church at South Chard.

There was no vicar or pastor, but a small man known as Uncle Sid, and his wife, Auntie Millie, who was not very small. They had been members of a local church that was very 'religious', but one day they had an encounter with God that changed everything. They were filled with the Spirit of God and started praising him, and praying to him, in a language they did not know – just like the church in the New Testament. They were asked to leave their church, rather like New Testament Christians having to leave the synagogue. They met together to worship in their home, and other people started joining them, so they built a 'chapel' in their garden, and when it was regularly full of people, they added an extension, and then a gallery. The people were not terribly middle-class, but ordinary local people. They expected the Lord to be in their meetings and they expected to see miracles. The praise almost shook the place, and especially when Auntie Millie 'played the swing doors' with her fists. There was no need for a drummer! We expected to sense the closeness of the living God in those meetings, and we were not disappointed. People were regularly converted and people were regularly healed. It was not so unusual for a celebrity to creep in, as they had heard about the place and what was happening there. One of the Beatles' wives turned up one evening, and probably thought that her husband's group was not so loud after all! There were several people in full-time ministry, and yet none of them was on a pay-roll, as they believed that the God who had called them, would meet their every need – and he did. From time to time there would be a collection, and it would be given to help support one of the 'ministers', but there were a lot of gifts from those who 'had' to those who were in need. I loved that place and I loved the people, and continue to stay in touch with many of them after more than forty years. Their denomination? They did not have one – they were just Christians.

A number of similar smaller churches had sprung up around the area, and I would sometimes visit them, and as there was rarely a scheduled 'speaker', would often share in the meeting what the Lord had recently been showing me from the Scriptures. And it was at one of those meetings that someone had a vision that was to change the course of our lives.

We had been in Shaftesbury for over four years, and were considering our future. We had been and looked at one or two practices, and also been offered a partnership where I was working. But we knew that the Lord would have a plan for our lives, and that there would be a recognizable peace when the next move was made clear – and we had not felt that peace yet. We considered several places and Norfolk in particular, and then someone had a vision. It was so clear, and they immediately shared it with the rest of us present. It was of a chessman, a knight, and Sheila and I felt that it could mean we were to move to Norfolk, as on a map, this would describe the way a knight would move from Dorset to Norfolk. That of course is very subjective, and we prayed with other people about the matter, and mentioned it to my parents. My father contacted our family dentist who had a colleague who was about to retire....... he would rather like a 'private sale.'

The practice in Norwich was run down, and the finance companies that boasted that they *always* helped dentists buy a practice, studied the practice records and told me that, sadly, this was the exception that proved the rule. My father had retired from the bank, but had worked with a fellow cashier, who was now a manager, so he took him out for a beer.... and he offered me a loan.

But I needed to raise some money myself, and so my fairly new Reliant Scimitar was sold for cash, and the local vicar's old estate car sat on my drive. It reeked of dog, but there was now money in the bank.

We were sad to leave that beautiful hilltop town, with its memories of our early-married life, birth of our first two daughters, and a scared patient hiding in a woodyard. And yet more wonderful serendipitous happenings awaited us in East Anglia, and if the woodyard incident had been somewhat unusual, I was still to experience the mystery of the Fox's glacier mint, the married couple who shared a set of false teeth, and a host of other characters who would enrich my life.

CHAPTER 8

The German, the Yank, and the Red-Haired Irishman – Locked in the Loo!

With patients streaming in to see several different dentists and hygienists working in multiple surgeries at the practice, reception staff would routinely ask the person checking in, "Which dentist do you see?"

"I see the young one." That was *me*!
"I see the old one." *That* was me!
"I see the German man." *That* too was me!
"I see the Yank." *That* was me!
"I see the red-haired Irishman." Even *that* was me!
"I see the lady with the long dark hair." That was Bob Williams! Bob often needed a haircut, and his voice would reach near falsetto tones when he was alarmed or excited.

Locked in the loo? I will come to that in a little while.

People's powers of observation are obviously impaired at times of emotional stress, but it was fascinating to hear these various descriptions of 'my dentist', though of little use to reception staff when it came to identifying which dentist the patient actually saw. So they would check through the appointment books. Today there are computers, and before that, we simply colour-coded the dentists. I had a green appointment book and green appointment cards, Bob was blue, Andy was red, Raymond was yellow and so on.

Ten years had passed since I had arrived in Norwich in my rather dilapidated Hillman Hunter estate, and wondered whether I really would make a living at the dental practice that finance companies would not touch with a barge pole.

Sheila and I may have believed that the Lord had directed us to buy this practice, and we certainly prayed together about 'getting it right' – but there were times when I would wake up in the night and ask myself if we had *really* heard God. My elderly predecessor had seen four patients in the morning and another four in the afternoon, and worked four days a week, and barely made a living. He had not needed much of an income – he had made his pile as a young man. My situation was different – I *was* a young man.

The practice building comprised two Victorian terraced houses knocked into one, and there was just one surgery that had been used, with a cast iron dental chair, and an old unit with a slow drill that had seen better days, bolted to one side, and a reconditioned fast drill on the other side. The waiting room had faded wallpaper and a few ancient dining chairs, and there was an office. Other rooms contained piles of dental magazines, and heaps of plaster of Paris models of teeth. It was damp and there were so few patients on the books.

I opened the front door of the practice just after New Year in 1974 – and patients almost stampeded in.

"Can you take me on?" and "I'm in agony," and "I've broken my false teeth," and "Please see me first – I'm dying of pain." Where had they all come from? How could so many people not have their own dentist to see?

I had taken on one girl, several months pregnant, to act as dental nurse and receptionist, and we both needed roller skates that first day. And the second. And the third, and so it continued, with there never being less than forty patients attending in a day.

People said it was amazing, and Christian friends said it was a miracle. Sheila and I felt it was both. In fact, three dentists in the city had retired that Christmas, and instead of selling their practices, they simply closed them and sold off the property. Thousands of people were left without a dentist, and word soon got round that I was open and ready for business. I had read in my Bible that the Lord likes to prosper his people, but this was overwhelming.

The bank had asked me to try to repay the loan in ten years, and I had asked for twenty-five. But with the number of patients flooding into the practice, I paid off the loan in ten months flat, and then went back and asked for another, in order to pay my tax bill on the first year's income, to add a second surgery and take on another dentist to help me. That was after the first year, and then after the second year I added a third surgery and took on another dentist. It was a further six years before I started building again, and added a fourth and fifth surgery and an education room, where we could teach children and adults about dental health. This was a loss-making exercise and somewhat *avant garde* at that time, but it enabled me to help the community of which I was a part.

The pregnant lady had worked with me for around three months before leaving and preparing for motherhood, so I then advertised for a receptionist and a nurse. Daphne joined the practice as receptionist, and was the main anchorperson for the fifteen or more years that I worked there. She then continued as receptionist for my successor. She was married to a farm manager in a small village just a few miles outside Norwich, and not only enjoyed engaging patients in conversation about families and holidays and such like, but was also knowledgeable about cows, horses and sugar beet!

The Eastern Daily Press is an excellent regional newspaper and widely read, though I myself had always read a national daily paper. But Daphne read the 'EDP' and would sometimes inform me that Mr. Smith would not be attending for his filling appointment on Thursday, or Mr. Jones would not be having his dentures fitted on Tuesday. "Cancelled has he?" I would remark.

"No," Daphne would reply, "He got three years for assault yesterday," or "He has just been sentenced to five years for burglary."

On occasions we would have a telephone call from a laboratory to tell us that some dentures or crowns would not be back when arranged, due to a power cut or similar, and we would have to cancel the patient.

"Mrs. Barker is not on the 'phone," one of the assistant receptionists would say with a worried expression.

"I'll 'phone Mrs. Bloggins," Daphne would say, and we would ask why. "Because she lives next door to Mrs. Hammond, and Mrs. Hammond is Mrs. Barker's cousin." She would explain.

"How on earth do you know *that*?" I would ask incredulously.

"I might talk a lot through the hatchway here all day," Daphne would say, almost defiantly, "But I am gathering useful information for the practice all the time, you know." Where would we have been without Daphne?!

Around a dozen different dentists worked as my associates during that time. They were mainly Christians, and I chose them, not just for their proficiency as dentists, but also for their warm and interesting personalities. I would periodically take them out for a lunch, or entertain them at my home for an evening, and the time was always filled with good humour and laughter. A number of them continue to be friends who I value enormously. In addition to the dentists, there were of course scores of nurses, and a few hygienists, nearly all of whom were appreciated by the patients and were great assets to the practice.

* * * * * * * * * *

The practice was just outside a large local authority housing estate where many people were unemployed, and most patients had their treatment free as they were on government benefits.

Someone told me that they had seen a large crowd of people standing round a car parked by the side of the road on the estate. "What's going on?" the man enquired. "Oh, they have found a car with a valid tax disc on the windscreen, and everyone's come to see what it looks like," was the response. It was perhaps a standing joke, but there could have been an element of truth in the story.

"I'm on Infidelity Benefit," said a middle-aged man, smiling benignly as he walked into my surgery.

"Infidelity Benefit?" I asked. I realized that the country had a left-wing government at that time, but to award people, even those who voted for them, for infidelity, seemed a benefit too far to me.

"Yes. I've been down the social offices, and they told me. Infidelity Benefit," he said softly, and sat down in the chair.

He had nothing in writing to that effect, but his general demeanour suggested he was on benefit of some description. The NHS was not run very tightly in those days, and so I wrote under the benefit section on the back of the dental form, "He says he is on Infidelity Benefit". My nurse was a local girl with the local dialect, and said that would give them a 'roight ole larf' at NHS HQ at Eastbourne.

But it happened again. "I'm on Infidelity Benefit," said a sad-looking balding man in a baggy grey suit that probably came from the local charity shop. "They told me down the social offices." And then another, and another. None of them seemed to be joking, and there was even a hint of pride that they actually *qualified* for their Infidelity Benefit.

I telephoned the local social security offices, where I was put through to the manager. He seemed a little embarrassed and assured me that there would be no more patients coming to me on 'Infidelity Benefit.' He paused, and then explained. They had taken on a new girl, who lived on the same estate as many of the claimants. Like them, she was 'not very good at words', and sometimes 'got them wrong.' She would take the details of the person claiming benefit, and carry them through to an assessor, who would decide what benefit the person was eligible for. And sometimes it was *Incapacity* Benefit – which could be considered as quite a long complicated word. The girl had not really come across that word before, but had heard people on television use one rather like it, and so went back to the claimant with "You're on Infidelity Benefit." In my mind I saw the claimant smiling and thanking the girl, and on returning home, telling his wife the good news – "I'm on Infidelity Benefit," and of his wife then leaning over the garden fence and telling her neighbour, "My Fred's on Infidelity Benefit", and of the neighbour saying, "Oh yes. There's several blokes on it down this road....." and so on.

I used to ask patients how often they cleaned their teeth, and they frequently seemed at a loss for words. "Once a day?" I would ask, and they would shake their head. "Every other day?" I would suggest, but they would tell me that it was not that often. The local doctor knew the people well, and had primed me. "What about Friday night?" I would say, and the patient would immediately look up with a bright smile. "Yes – Friday night!" would be the response. Friday was the day those in work were paid, and Friday night was when everybody went to the local pub. So they brushed their teeth on Friday night. Simple.

Another matter that caused me some concern, was the fact that it was not uncommon for a family of five or six people to share just one toothbrush. I was speaking to the local doctor about it, and of the potential for cross infection among those who used it. "Don't worry about it, old chap," he reassured me. "They *share* the toothbrush, but nobody actually *uses* it."

One morning a couple came into my surgery together. The rather well-fed lady was the spokesperson, while her husband, who seemed dwarfed beside her, gave support by repeating the last few words of her previous sentence.

"We were wondering whether we qualify for new teeth," she volunteered.

"Teeth," said the husband.

"We'd really like some new teeth, on the 'Nash," she continued.

"On the 'Nash." He wanted to make absolutely certain they would be treated on the National Health Service.

"We wanted to know if we qualify. Both of us," she continued.

"Both of us," he said by way of emphasis.

I asked them how long they had been wearing their false teeth (though they looked as if they had forgotten to put them in that day), and also whether they were in discomfort with them.

They looked at each other blankly, and then the spokesperson said, "Actually, we share a set."

"A set," came the echo.

I asked how long they had shared a set of teeth, and they could not remember. I asked which of them the dentures actually belonged to, but they could not remember whether they were his, hers, or someone else's, as it had been a long time now. I enquired whether they ate their meals in relays, and they looked completely blank, before the wife said, "I suppose so," and her husband simply nodded.

One month later they both marched out through my front door, and both – *both* – were smiling at the world.

I will always remember a man who had a rather messy story to tell, and who rendered it particularly tedious by interjecting "You know how it is?" when I most certainly did not. He entered the surgery appearing rather agitated, and it was obvious that he had no teeth in his mouth, as his cheeks had fallen in and his chin was almost bouncing off the underside of his nose when he closed his mouth.

"I want some new teef," he slurred, obviously not used to speaking without them. I lothst them yetherday. You know how it is."

"I'll have a look at your mouth, and then take some impressions," I explained.

But he had to tell me all about it, and using words that I would rather not repeat. Well, they were not obscene, but simply not very nice!

"I was goin' through the centre of Norwich on a bus, you see, upstairs, and I got this pain in my (stomach)" he continued, though he used a rather vulgar word for stomach. "You know how it is."

In fact it was a long time since I had travelled on a bus, and did not know how it was, and nor had I had a pain in my stomach on one, and so I did not know how that was either. But for the sake of other patients waiting to see me –

"Yes, yes, of course," I replied, and picked up my mouth mirror.

"Well, I knew the pain wasn't goin' to get better, and that I was goin' to (vomit). You know how it is?" he said, with a very earnest look.

"Let's have a look at your gums," I almost pleaded, but to no avail.

"I didn't want to (vomit) all over the top of the bus, did I? Not nice. So I stuck my head out of the window."

I did not realize that buses had windows that you could stick your head out of, and could not help asking, "In the centre of Norwich? Where everyone is shopping?"

"Yes mate. I wasn't going to do it all over the seats in the bus, was I? So I stuck my head out. You know how it is?"

"Of course. Yes, I'm sure. So you would like some new teeth?"

"Well, I stuck my head out the window, and I done it. But when I'd finished, my teeth were gone. Gone!" he said with a look that told me I should look truly amazed.

"Amazing," I said on cue.

"So what I done was, I waited till the next stop, and then I got off and ran back to where I'd done it. All over the pavement it was, mate. But you know what? Someone had had 'em."

Before proceeding to examine his mouth and take impressions, I could not help but ask this man an important question.

"What number bus do you travel through the city centre on?" I enquired.

"Number 23," he replied, and I made a mental note of it, because if I saw that bus approaching while I was walking through the city, I would most certainly withdraw into a shop doorway. I now knew how it was – or at least, how it could be!

Shared toothbrushes, shared dentures, infidelity benefit, vomiting from buses – there seemed no end to the variety of incidents and stories that caused me to smile, either at the time or later whilst reflecting on them. Another happening that might have evoked a degree of anger in some, only caused me to smile broadly, and still does.

A lady of great girth clad in a rainproof coat of greater girth entered the front door, passed straight through the waiting room and into the patient's toilet. A man sitting in the waiting area got up and walked over to reception.

"You need to watch her," he said, and returned to his seat.

Around ten minutes later the lady emerged from the toilet, and walked slowly and awkwardly towards the front door again, and on reaching it appeared to have difficulty in holding the handle and opening it. One of the receptionists went over to assist, but the lady did not notice this, and continued fumbling with the door handle. Suddenly there was a tremendous clatter as two bottles of lavatory cleaner, some cans of air-freshener and a few toilet rolls crashed out from under her coat and rolled around the floor. She smiled sweetly at reception and slipped out through the door, leaving the objects strewn across the hall.

"Told you to watch her," said the man in the waiting room. Rather like Whitechapel, many people knew each other within this community.

But I loved the people from that area. There was a 'warmth' about most of them, and 'what you saw was what you got.' I enjoyed conversation with them, and occasionally I would be invited round for a cup of tea, and sometimes I would accept.

There was rarely a problem with payment, as so many were on government benefits. I could not carry out treatment in the manner that I had been trained at the London, or I would have gone bankrupt within six months, but I treated them to the very best of my ability within the confines of the NHS. Life is not about money – it is God's world and God's people, and I found fulfilment in enjoying their company and doing what I could for them.

* * * * * * * * * *

Having my own practice had put me on a steep learning curve. My predecessor had told me never to leave money or gold crowns on the premises, and to expect a visit from one of the local burglars before too long. However, he assured me, once the first one had made his call, word would go round the other villains, "Lawrence takes the money home." But it seemed that no one had told the local underworld fraternity that this was the way it worked.

Around three or four months after opening, I arrived one morning to find a rear window slightly open, and every cupboard door and every drawer open. Chummy had paid us his visit! I called the police and the local CID came round, dusted for fingerprints and made lots of notes. "Professional job sir," said the more senior of the two. "Every drawer opened just far enough to take a good look. They start from the bottom and work up, so there's no time lost closing them." As nothing had been taken, I assumed that the professional villain would make sure that every other villain was told, "Lawrence takes the money home." But somehow he forgot.

It was Easter 1982 and I was coordinating a convention in Norwich for the evangelist Don Double. I took time off from the surgery, and usually left the convention site quite late. One evening I decided to call in at my surgery to catch up on a little paperwork, and as I unlocked the front door and entered the hall, I was vaguely aware of a light showing for a second under the office door. I was going to work in the office anyway, and opened the door and put the light on, and there crouching in the corner of the room was - a villain! I stared at him, but did not quite believe what I was seeing. There should not be anybody here in the office... what was this man doing?... and suddenly I realised and froze.

I felt that I needed to appear strong and assertive, and so with my heart almost audibly thumping, I said loudly, "Just what do you think you're doing here?"

"You've got me, mate," said the man in black. No doubt black shoes, black trousers, black polo neck pullover, and short black, probably dyed, hair was all part of the uniform.

"You've got me mate, got me," said the terrified villain. I had read a few crime stories as a boy, and back in the late 1950s had observed that villains always said, "OK guv, it's a fair cop." Obviously times were changing!

But what should I do with the chap? "I'll show you how I got in," said my prisoner, and led me through to the patient's toilet. "That winder mate - easy."

My brain was working overtime. If I telephoned the police, would he fight... run... break the place up? After a minute's silent thought I decided to let the man go.

"This time I am going to let you go," I told him, walking to the front door, opening it wide and standing back. And suddenly he was gone, running like a hare along the poorly lit main road on which my practice stood.

Had I done the right thing? Of course, after the event one always knows better. I had a number of policemen as patients, and the first one I told uttered words that I would never use, let alone print. But another older and wiser officer was more sanguine.

"Well sir," he said in a voice that reminded me of Dixon of Dock Green, "Discretion is the better part of valour." I was not sure what he meant by this, and he read my puzzled expression. "Might 'ave 'ad a knife. You never know. Discretion's the better part of valour; that's what I always say," he explained, which made me feel a lot better.

So I had a burglar alarm fitted, and felt I could now relax in the evenings. However, that was not to be, and after a couple of months my telephone rang at around 10 p.m. and a policeman informed me that my alarm was ringing and he would meet me at the surgery. It was a very short drive away, and soon I met two uniformed officers, who had a small audience on the pavement in front of Lockett's Fish and Chip Shop opposite the surgery. The alarm was echoing harshly along the brick buildings on either side of the road as I unlocked the front door, and the three of us trooped in. There was no one to be seen as we searched the premises from top to bottom, and one of the officers asked if I could unlock the rear door so that he could search the back garden.

As soon as the door was opened there was an unmistakable aroma - cod and chips! This villain was prepared to be patient as he worked on forcing open the rear door to the premises, and had had the forethought to take with him, not cod and chips, but *double* cod and chips, which was sitting on the doorstep and still warm. Needless to say the police went to the fish and chip shop across the road and enquired, "Do you recall anyone ordering double cod and chips here this evening, sir?"

"Maybe fifty, or perhaps sixty," was the reply. "Like a description officer?"

* * * * * * * * * *

We had arrived back in Norfolk at the end of 1973, and when we moved into our first house in the city of Norwich, a very modest little detached house within cycling distance of the practice, Sheila was heavily pregnant with our third child. Naomi was born that June, and again I could not believe how beautiful she was.

I had met a few other Christians who had started meeting in a home, and we joined them on Sundays. We thought that there would be the freedom for God to move amongst us that we had experienced in the church near Chard, but in fact the meetings were quite organized. The room they met in was of modest proportions, and although we lived in a small house, there was virtually just one room downstairs, which gave us space. The meetings moved to our home, and I learned to play a few chords on the guitar – and we praised the Lord! Did we! The numbers started to grow, and after eighteen months or so there were around seventy people sitting shoulder to shoulder across the floor, and sometimes outside in the small hall, and even up the stairs. I would start to strum and sing praises to God, and it was as if the entire assembly stood up *en bloc* (maybe they were stuck together with the heat) and the house would resonate with singing, clapping and foot tapping. People were converted to Christ, some were miraculously healed, prayers were answered, and Sheila and I found ourselves so very busy. People wanted to come and talk through their problems and situations, or for us to pray together with them, or just listen. There were meetings for church leaders – and all with three children and later, a fourth on the way. Although I liked my work and loved my patients, I reduced my working week at the practice to, first four days, and then three, but there was immense stress in our lives. One of the other leaders had a very different approach to church than Sheila and me, and we spent a lot of time trying to see things his way, though not wanting to compromise on what we saw in scripture. These days were some of the happiest, but also some of the most difficult.

* * * * * * * * *

I had also started doing something altogether new to me within the field of dentistry – domiciliary work. Like most dentists, I would periodically receive a request to go to some-one's home because they needed new dentures but were house-bound. I would take a bag of impression material, trays and other necessary items to where they lived, and carry out the treatment. It was not easy, and sometimes I would find that something I needed had been left at the practice. Also, the NHS fee for travelling to the patient was a positive disincentive, and it all took so much time.

And yet, here was a great need within the local community and across the region. People with nervous breakdowns, agoraphobia, muscular dystrophy, multiple sclerosis, arthritis and a host of other conditions could not get to the dentist, and often suffered in silence. With several other dentists now working at the practice, I felt I could afford to spend one day a week making a loss, but helping the needy.

I held office in the British Dental Association in our area, and let it be known amongst colleagues that I was prepared to travel and would carry out whatever treatment I could. The majority of the work was making new dentures, but I obtained a portable dental drill unit, and even carried out cosmetic crowns on one patient sitting in an armchair. Whilst drilling, the nurse would squirt the tooth with a multi-shot water pistol to stop it from overheating! And everything was under the NHS.

There were unforeseen difficulties at times. On one occasion I rang the doorbell of the house where the patient lived, and it was answered, not by the wife as was usually the case, but by a younger lady.

"Are you the undertaker?" asked the daughter of the recently deceased. Another 'unfinished treatment', and perhaps a factor contributing to one of our friends in the church asking me one day, "How are those homicidals going?" Domiciliaries, homicidals..... another gentleman who was 'not very good at words!'

On another occasion I was asked to visit Ethel, a lady of ninety-two, married to Frank, who was ninety-three. They lived in a little wooden house on the banks of the river Wensum that flows through Norwich. Frank had worked most of his life with boats, and they had known each other since she was three and he was four. She had worn the same false teeth since she was twenty – a total of seventy-two years! They were transparent in places, and had cracked.

I checked her mouth, and then took the lower impression, after which the nurse mixed up impression material for the upper. When I removed the upper impression, there was a Fox's glacier mint stuck in the middle of it.

"Where did this come from?" I enquired. But she was deaf, and though I shouted and gesticulated, it was to no avail. Could I possibly have missed it whilst inspecting the mouth? Surely not. Or did she deftly flick it in whilst I was picking up the impression tray? I doubt that too. And so the 'Mystery of the Fox's Glacier Mint' will remain a mystery – but I still sometimes think about it.

After about 4 visits the dentures were finished and I called round and fitted them. I did two follow-up visits to adjust them a little, and all seemed well. However, six weeks after fitting the teeth, Ethel fell out of bed one night, and only survived a day or two. Her daughter telephoned the practice and thanked me for what I had done and told me the sad news. I waited a couple of weeks, and then drove round to the little house on the river bank, and had a cup of tea with Frank. He told me they had been married over seventy-five years, and with tears welling up in his eyes, smiled and said, "The Lord has always been good to us." As I walked back to my car there were tears in my eyes too.

Whilst the most common request from house-bound patients was for new false teeth, the greatest need was for company. These people were lonely, and after fitting the new dentures, I would be called back week after week, and always offered a cup of tea for which I just did not have time. So I decided that I would set aside a day for visiting lonely domiciliary patients and drinking tea, leaving around 30 minutes for each visit and planning it so that a ten minute drive would take me from house to house.

By mid-morning my bladder was fairly bursting, and I asked a lady if I could use her toilet. Following her directions I found the loo, and as I locked the door heard the most ominous rattling and clunking sound. After flushing I tried the door, but it would not unlock, and I banged loudly on the door. The loo was entirely internal with no window, and the patient was deaf, of course, as well as being severely arthritic. I shouted. I banged. Eventually I heard footsteps slowly approaching, and a shaky voice enquired, "Are you alright?" Of course I wasn't, and I shouted out that I was locked in. "The lock's faulty," she volunteered, and I banged on the door again. "I'll get a handyman," said the lady, and I could hear her slowly shuffling down the hallway. It seemed an age before the handyman arrived – because it *was* an age. "Out you come," he said, grinning as he eventually opened the door for me. And out I came – the German, the Yank, the red-haired Irishman, the young man, the old man...... and now I was the distressed and dishevelled man.

Just to the north of Norwich in a small village remarkably-named Stratton Strawless, was a park for mobile homes, mainly static caravans. This became a regular destination for me on my domiciliary days. It was back in the mid to late 1970s, and at that time the lanes on which the 'vans were situated were made of cinders, broken bricks and rubble rolled flat, whilst the caravans themselves had generally seen far better days.

Having received a request for a visit from a couple of ladies who shared a caravan and who 'wanted teeth', I found myself knocking on their front door. It was opened by a lady with long dark straggly hair, and a gaunt look betraying a total lack of teeth. Aged in her mid-thirties, she could have passed for late fifties, and a black cat and a broomstick would not have seemed out of place. Her mother was around twenty years her senior in years and in looks. I examined their mouths and took impressions to start the denture-making process, and was asked if I would like coffee while I sat and wrote up records for two new patients. This seemed an excellent idea, until it was placed in front of me - in a one pint NAAFI beer mug! That was quite a long visit.

Winter had definitely arrived, with a few inches of snow on the ground by the time I returned for the fourth visit, to fit the dentures. Such weather brought out the child in me, and my children and I had our own toboggans - theirs and mine. We would take them up to Mousehold Heath, which boasted some of the very few tobogganable slopes to be found in the city.

The snow made the garden look tidy, by concealing so much. But snow was also revealing, in that some members of staff would be 'unable to get there' whilst others *always* arrived. And in this matter, distance was nothing to do with it. I can remember a severe weather warning being followed by a significant fall of snow, and yet a doctor and his daughter arrived early for an appointment, having driven fifty miles from Hunstanton, whereas many local people 'couldn't possibly get in.' One patient back in Shaftesbury had arrived on horseback in such weather.

So I drove out to 'Woodland View' at Stratton Strawless and fitted the two sets of dentures, and having declined a pint of coffee, climbed back into my Daimler, forgetting that snow can conceal such things as the edge of the road. In doing a three point turn outside their caravan, my best guess was wrong, and having sunk into the snow-covered mud at least to my axles, I found myself back in their home, drinking a pint of coffee as we awaited a tractor to come and pull me out. That would not happen today as, nearly forty years on, the site has been transformed into a smart little village where a small number of our friends make their home.

My domiciliary days were not without their trials and tribulations, being locked in a toilet, having my car stuck in thawing snow and underlying mud, finding my shoes so often sticking to the carpets that had been 'leaked on' for months, and being head-butted by small dogs, frustrated at the lack of exercise from their owners incarceration. In addition to this, I probably made a financial loss in carrying out such work under the National Health Service. But I felt that those days were of significant benefit to people in the local community, and there was a great sense of fulfilment in carrying out their treatment over many years.

* * * * * * * * * *

Life now revolved around the family, the practice, the church, and an occasional game of squash to try and keep fit. We had four daughters by now, as Deborah had joined us. Not only was she another incredibly beautiful baby, but also she had her father's rather distinctive hair.

Life was hectic, and I just could not cope. My personal life became extremely muddled, and I hated myself for not coping, and struggled to keep everything together – my health, my family, and my work. The church? – the small gathering that had been in our home had grown, moved into a community centre, and then gone on to number several hundred. I had been doing far too much, and as a family we had decided to join a more conventional church where that side of life would be less demanding for a while.

If I found it difficult to cope with life, Sheila had a worse time trying to cope with me whilst also looking after four children, and the result was that we ended up separated. I shed many tears, and I am sure the rest of the family did too. I wonder at times how people outside the family of God manage to come through some of the crises of life. I spent time daily, as I had since I had first become a Christian, reading the scriptures and finding strength and encouragement, and immersing myself in the presence of God in prayer. A Christian family in a nearby town offered me accommodation. They were a tremendous support to me at that time while I tried to get the marriage back together - unsuccessfully.

It seemed as if life had almost come to an end, but my reading of Scripture tells me that the person who seeks to walk with God through this life has a more glorious future than their past ever was. I was not to know that just seven miles away was a small country cottage clad in red roses, just waiting for me. Nor could I have guessed of two areas of business that were yet to open up for me, and which would be described by a local newspaper as 'Heaven and Hell'. And if I had known in advance that twice within a month I would find myself staring at a used needle sticking out of the end of my finger – a needle infected with Hepatitis C and probably HIV.......... but these delights and challenges were soon to arrive.

CHAPTER 9

Heaven and Hell, a Murder, and a Comedian!

"Heaven and Hell exist side by side," read a local newspaper in an article on the fact that I had a Christian bookshop and a dental practice next door to each other in a Norfolk market town.

"But which is which?" quipped a friend of mine from the local church.

I had stayed with the family in that town for six months, but could not stay there forever. Their friends were so supportive and friendly to me, and three couples had promised to pray together daily that the marriage would be restored, until either it *did* come together or became clear that it would not.

Although my prayer was for the restoration of marriage and family, I felt I needed to take steps in case I was unsuccessful in this. I had always dreamed of living in an older property out in the country, and so went to every estate agent I could find and asked to be informed of anything suitable that came on the market. However, all I received related to modern properties and city properties. In addition to this, I had very little money, as I had invested so much in the Norwich practice and was supporting my wife and children to live in the manner to which they had been accustomed. I decided that I would settle for anything – but it had to be inexpensive.

And having decided to stop looking for that beautiful country cottage, I opened the local newspaper and there, right in front of my eyes, was a beautiful country cottage for sale.

No estate agents had sent me details, and so I found out where it was and went to see the vendors.

It was pink, though I preferred to call it 'rose', and the trellis holding the multitude of red roses on the front wall almost smiled at me as I walked across the lawn. Having been shown around, I immediately made an offer for the property, only to be told by the lovely couple whose home it had been for the past thirty-three years that after being on the market for just one week, my offer was the fourth – and the lowest. However, they smiled at me and said that if I would but raise my offer just a little, they would sell to me, even though it would still be the lowest, as I had nowhere to sell and could proceed immediately with the purchase. It was agreed.

There was another problem though, in that I had virtually no savings and there was a mortgage famine. The result of money being so tight in the summer of 1983 resulted in people not being able to obtain a 100% mortgage, and also having to wait for three months in a 'mortgage queue'. I explained this to George and Maisie who were selling the cottage, and they said they knew of a building society that might be helpful.

The following day I received a telephone call from a man who introduced himself as manager of a small building society of which I had not heard before. I told him that the vendors and I had agreed a certain price for the sale of the cottage, but that I had not got savings on which to draw for a deposit.

"You can have a 100% loan," replied the building society manager.

"That's amazing," I responded. "I understood from everything I read in the newspapers that no banks or building societies would give more than 80% loans, and usually less than that."

"Absolutely right," said the manager, "but George and Maisie are my parents and I want to see that they are alright."

"O.K. Thanks," I said, "But there is a three month queue before any money can be made available, is there not?"

"Absolutely right," said the manager, "but George and Maisie are my parents and I want to see that they are alright. You can have it tomorrow if you like!"

"Thank you again," I replied, "but you know nothing about me. Surely you cannot simply offer me the money in this way."

"I know *everything* about you," said the manager. "George and Maisie are my parents and I have done my homework on you!"

Maybe George and Maisie were being looked after by their son, but I most certainly felt that I was being looked after by my Father. And as I have gone through life I have found time and time again, that when the odds seem stacked against me, it is as though a divine hand reaches down and changes things. My Norwich practice was described by a finance company as a 'dead duck', and yet I had paid off a ten-year loan in ten months. When I was out of my home and trying to cope in rented rooms, a family I hardly knew came and offered me accommodation. They also cooked for me, and never charged me a penny. And now there was the cottage, and the loan, and the arrangements for it. These things are what I believe the sceptics call 'coincidences'. I love them – and praise God for them!

I bought the cottage in May 1983, but continued to live with the family a few miles away. If I could get the marriage together, Sheila and I could keep the cottage as a holiday home, or we could sell it. But the marriage did not come together, and I moved in at the beginning of September that year. It was seven miles from my new friends in the town, and the same from my practice in the city. More importantly, it was only four miles from my old family home, which I was making over to Sheila, and so the children were really close. On occasions they would cycle over to see me, and we spent time together as often as we could.

I had never cooked, but spent what little money I had on putting in a simple kitchen (the existing one was antiquated) and a bathroom. There had been a bath, washbasin and toilet behind a screen at the back of the kitchen, but I wanted something a little better for my daughters. And there were two bedrooms – one for me, and one for them.

With the cooker came a cookbook, and it started at my level with instructions for boiling a potato – but before very long I was giving three course dinner parties for around half a dozen people, and though I often produced boeuf bourguignon, goulash or beef stroganoff, my favourite dishes were curries and chillies. I even started making my own curry powder, using various spices, which I ground together in an electric coffee grinder. My friends said they loved the curry, but the coffee blew their heads off! Well, my taste in curry was vindaloo.

At the top of the garden I cleared some ground and drove in stakes to which I attached chicken netting. The hens seemed to do well, and so I got a cockerel and bred them. This all seemed like fun during what was still, at times, a rather depressing period in my life. So I launched out further and kept ducks. There was also a degree of nostalgia, in that my parents had kept chickens when I was young, and when I went to collect the eggs the smell of the warm straw would take me back to those idyllic days of childhood many decades earlier.

One year later there was the opportunity to buy some property in a side street away from the town centre, a few hundred yards from the house where the kind Christian people had accommodated me the previous year. I immediately felt this was divinely planned for me, and although my accountant told me there was a 50% likelihood of it bankrupting me, I took out a large loan and started a part-time practice there. A lady called Dawn, who had worked at my Norwich practice some years earlier, became my nurse and receptionist.

The property was larger than I needed for a small dental practice, and six months after opening, I used part of the premises to open a Christian bookshop. This seemed so foolhardy to my accountant that he told me to name it 'Suicide' – I have written more about this in another book, which also chronicles several other ways in which my life has been marked by miraculous intervention. Needless to say perhaps, the practice prospered to such an extent that I added a second surgery for another associate dentist that first year, and later took on a dental hygienist and added a third surgery. The bookshop made a profit some years, but usually a loss, and yet was open for just under twenty years. So many lives were touched by it.

* * * * * * * * * *

The new practice had a great 'family' feel to it, and I would regularly take the staff out to lunch to show appreciation for their hard work and cheerfulness. And the years flew by as I just loved my country home and the market town practice. And what of the Norwich practice? I sold it to my senior associate, and he expanded it still further. He too is a Christian dentist with four children, and he is currently *my* dentist. He is a drummer in his church, and I am a guitar player in mine.

Romance blossomed between Dawn and me, and after a few years we married. We enjoyed living in the cottage, though we extended it over the years, and we also made a good team at the practice. In addition to this, we were very active members of a church in the town that grew from nearly thirty of us to around three hundred in a very short period of time.

* * * * * * * * * *

It was a Monday morning and the weekend's dental casualties were descending on us. "I've lost my dentures," said a middle-aged man forlornly, and then proceeded to tell me in great detail exactly what had happened.

Every year, thousands of people lose their false teeth, and the ways in which they do so are multitudinous. Some of the ways in which they were lost we heard over and over again, and yet sometimes there would be something new.

The most common way of losing false teeth? "They went down the toilet, mate," were words we heard so many times. When I first started in practice, 'dentures down the loo' was something that happened mostly in late winter, because that was when sickness was going around. As time passed, it seemed to be something that occurred all year round. In fact, there is usually a bug (it never used to be called a 'bug') going round, and it is usually named after some part of the anatomy – the 'tummy' bug, the 'throat' bug, the 'head' bug and so on. But it was predominantly late winter when people would telephone the practice and try and tell us (speaking could be a little difficult without teeth) that they had lost their teeth.

"I ran to the loo, and after I'd flushed it, I realized they'd gone," was a recurring message. The receptionist would come in and say, "There's another one just 'phoned up!"

A telephonist telephoned us to say that she had just dropped her teeth on the floor and they had shattered. She was very difficult to understand, and we did not hold out much hope of her keeping her job. But in these situations we would telephone the technicians, who would accelerate the process, even under the NHS. Everyone tried to be as understanding as possible.

Everybody who wears false teeth should have a spare set in case of loss, and I would tell this to all my patients. I wear spectacles and always have a spare pair to hand, and likewise patients with false teeth should be prepared for the worst.

Another recurring theme went something like this. "Can you see my mother please? She has lost her teeth, and she can't find them anywhere. She hasn't been too well recently, and has just been sitting in an armchair by the fire. She would take her teeth out each day, as she found it more relaxing to sit without them, and she would put them on a tissue on the arm of the chair. She would also use tissues to wipe her mouth, and then place those on the arm of the chair. Every now and again one of us would throw all the old tissues on the fire.........."

And then there was the young man who came in after a New Year's party. "Hey mate, can you make me some new teef? You see, I went to a party New Year's Eve – great party with lots of booze and lots of women. Fantastic mate – I can't remember too much about the evening really, and – well," (starting to snigger), "I'm not going to tell you where I woke up the next morning," (further sniggering), "but my teeth – gone they were. Haven't a clue where I lost them or where they might be. So can you do me some teef, mate?"

On another occasion a glum looking lady produced the remains of a denture, which was basically the pink palate that covered the roof of the mouth, and with around three teeth on it. All the front part was missing, and there was a ragged edge.

"The dog got 'em!" she sighed.

"Then it's a good job you weren't wearing them at the time," I replied. She nodded.

A variation on a theme was, "They found them in the shrubbery, but they're damaged." The lady telling me was a resident at a home for the elderly a few hundred yards from the practice, and was famous there for complaining about, well.... everything, so we were told. She had started to become preoccupied with her false teeth, and spoke about them all day long, every day, and to everyone. And then another resident could stand it no more, and seeing them on the arm of the lady's chair, she snatched them, and hobbled off with the edentulous one in not-so-hot pursuit. On reaching a window, she opened it and hurled the offending articles as far as she could, saying "That will shut you up." The staff formed a search party and found them in the shrubbery, and the lady brought in the rather damaged items for repair.

A young middle-aged man sat in the chair one day and said, "I must tell you what happened to me and my teeth this summer." I had the time, and it seemed he was determined to tell me anyway, and his story went like this.

"We decided that we were going to take our family to the seaside this year, for a traditional British beach holiday – sand

and sea, just like when we were young. So we booked into our hotel, and as the sun was shining, we went down to the beach and I was soon swimming along parallel with the shore. I noticed something in the sea ahead of me and thought it was a fish, but when I actually saw what it was – Heck, it was my false teeth, doing the breaststroke and going faster than I was! I swam with all my might, but they just vanished into the sea ahead of me. I was devastated, and told my wife that I was not going to be seen without teeth, and would be spending the rest of the week in our hotel room reading. But later I had an idea, and under cover of darkness, I slipped out of the hotel and crept along the high tide line. And there amongst the seaweed - I found them, both upper and lower! They were definitely mine, because they fitted so well. So I enjoyed the rest of the holiday, and took them out when swimming after that."

Over the years I have done a significant amount of public speaking, ranging from Bible teaching and evangelistic addresses, to simple after-dinner speaking as entertainment to make people laugh. I started with the Women's Institute where I got a cup of tea and a biscuit, and graduated up to dinners given by political parties where I was sent the rather posh menu in advance in order to select what I would like to eat. I sometimes mention the man whose dentures did the breaststroke, and occasionally someone will approach me afterwards and suggest the story was not true. But on two occasions someone has come up to me and told me that the same thing had happened to them. So there are at least three people I have met who have experienced this.

There is another story I have frequently been told, and about which I do have doubts. Every nurse is told this story, and I have someone approach me and relate the tale at around two out of three meetings where I speak on the subject. It goes like this: "When I was training to be a nurse I was told about a new girl working on the ward who was told to collect the false teeth from each of the patients there. Well, she went round with a bowl and put them all in it, and then – she didn't know which teeth belonged to which patient! So we were told we should always take the teeth out individually and keep them separate." Maybe you have already heard that story.

* * * * * * * * * *

When I started the new practice I had told people that it was not a branch practice, but a 'twig' practice, because it was so small. But it rapidly became a thriving and mature practice, and one day I received a telephone call from a local rehabilitation centre for drug addicts asking if I could see some of their clients. They had been to several other practices, but been shown the door. I said I would treat them for a few hours a week, and keep any contract with them under review.

Many of these people had come straight from prison to the centre – they had been sentenced for burglary, theft, prostitution and such like, as they had needed cash to finance their addiction. There were also successful businessmen and other professionals – and they were great people. I was called 'mate' and 'darlin', and when I introduced myself as 'Barrie' and simply chatted with them about my days in London while the Kray brothers were so busy, it was as though barriers came down and we were friends for life. I admired so many of those people for tackling their addictive habits, but sadly, many relapsed.

Cindy had been on heroin, but now felt she was free of it. She spoke about addiction with both intelligence and clarity, and clearly had a deep understanding of the problem. I asked her what she was going to do when she had finished the course, and she said she was going to become a counselor in order to help others. I asked her what she had done in the past, and she said, "You don't want to know!" Then she added, "I was on the streets, wasn't I." She looked forward to launching into a new life and a career helping others – but relapsed in less than a year.

Another young lady, Josie, had come straight to Norfolk from Holloway Prison in London, and I enjoyed conversations with her. She was an intelligent lady, not unattractive except for a few missing teeth for which I obtained permission from the NHS to carry out bridgework. One day she pulled up her trouser leg and said, "What do you think this is?"

I was tempted to say, "Your leg, Josie," but noticed that she was pointing to a band around her ankle.

"It's a tag," she explained. "In two days' time they will take it off, and I will get my little baby back that they took from me when I went to prison." She was understandably excited at having her child back, and I felt really happy for her.

A few days later her photograph was on the front page of the national newspapers and television news programmes. The day before the tag was to be removed, she had cut it off and absconded from the centre. Meeting up with an old flame, they set out to obtain enough cash to finance a drug addiction that cost £300 a day. Josie had told me in the surgery that she was an ace at stealing handbags, and this is what she was doing to pay for their drugs. However, one lady whose bag she stole started chasing her, and jumping back into the car they had stolen, her boyfriend had driven at the lady and killed her. They both appeared at the Old Bailey where Josie received a sentence of further time in prison for the handbag theft, while her boyfriend was found guilty of manslaughter, though I would have thought it was murder.

Did others manage to get free of their addiction and stay free? I only saw these people for their dental treatment, but I hope that many did. I really liked the people.

Many of them had hepatitis C, and others HIV. A number with HIV would not even know they were infected, and all patients are treated by dentists as if they have every disease known to man - because they might.

One day I had found that a young lady from the centre needed more treatment than I had anticipated, and as a result, I was running several minutes late. After she had left the surgery, I helped the nurse to clear the work surfaces and prepare the surgery for the next patient. And suddenly – OUCH! I thought that I had placed all the used needles in the sharps container, but had carelessly overlooked one, and now it was sticking out of the end of my finger. The patient had been a prostitute before attending the centre, and had tested hepatitis C positive, and very possibly HIV too. I withdrew the needle, and tried to make my finger bleed as much as possible, though I knew that the viruses that cause these diseases die fairly quickly once out of the body. However, I also knew that hepatitis C was extremely infectious, much more than the hepatitis B that we had all been warned about so much at dental school. As a result of the needle stick injury, I had to report to a blood-testing centre in Norwich for tests, first weekly and then less frequently for a year. And then, almost unbelievably, I did exactly the same thing again within a month, and so was back at the blood-testing centre faster than anticipated. I was eventually declared to be clear, but this is just one of those risks one takes when volunteering to treat high-risk patients.

A short sequel to the above incident was that some years later I was relating to a patient what had happened with the needle stick injury, and recalled how on seeing the needle sticking out of the end of my finger, I had said, "Oh no!"

The patient, on hearing this, looked at the nurse and, grinning, said, "I don't think Dr. Lawrence really said "*Oh No*", did he?"

The nurse thought for a moment, and said, "Actually, that *is* what he said." But it would have been rather easy to have let something else slip out, if I had been in the habit of using different words!

* * * * * * * * *

There was also an event, which we jokingly said 'made us famous'. We had a new trainee nurse at the practice, a fellow called Frank. He came under a training scheme, and the organization that ran it decided to advertise on television. They asked if they could use the surgery, and whether I would be prepared to be filmed with Frank 'starring' as nurse. We agreed, and there was great excitement as cameramen and lighting were brought into the surgery. My receptionist asked if she could be 'the patient' and had her hair nicely styled, and one of the other nurses had asked if she could be 'the patient' and had her hair nicely styled too.

Hot on the heels of the cameramen and crew came the director, a lady who announced, "I'm going to be 'the patient.'" So that was settled!

I always wore a pinstriped suit and bow tie for my work, and was wearing my smartest polka dot one for the film. Someone told us to get ready, and then shouted something like 'Take' and I went into the director's open mouth with mirror and probe. I couldn't resist saying from behind my mask, "These teeth are absolutely *awful*," at which the director pushed me away and creased up laughing. So we started again, even though it was 'silent', and after an hour or so they had three different sequences ready for their advert.

That advert was shown on Anglia Television night after night for nearly a year, and after a short break appeared yet again for a further run. Also patients would come into the surgery and say they had seen me on the screen at the cinema in Norwich, where the advert was running just prior to the showing of the film, 'The English Patient'. Each of the three sequences lasted for around one second, and was one of a batch that were shown – but we told people we were famous!

There is one other little incident that always makes me smile when I remember it. I had a patient who was a professional singer and comedian, and a very good one at that. Johnny Cleveland had been coming to the surgery for many years and one day had to attend for an extraction. Realising that the young trainee nurse on reception was new, he asked, "Excuse me, but I'm having a tooth out this afternoon. Will I be able to play the piano this evening?" Frank immediately reassured him, with "No problem at all with that. You can certainly play the piano this evening."

"Absolutely amazing," said Johnny, "I've always wanted to play the piano." Frank found this all very strange and worrying and came through and told me about it!

* * * * * * * * * *

Many years had passed since I had given that 'first injection' and carried out that 'first filling', and retirement had now appeared over the horizon. The children had grown up, and after supporting their mother in addition to my daughters for nearly twenty years, it seemed that we might be able to open up the leisure side of our lives a little more, as well as maybe doing more work for the church. One of my daughters had come to live with us after she left University, but was now working in the Midlands, and another daughter was based with us, though studying for much of the year at Cambridge University.

A cruise from Southampton, across the Atlantic to the Caribbean, and then on to Venezuela had been Dawn's preferred way of celebrating retirement, and we started looking at such adventures in travel brochures.

And then suddenly, and for me, totally unexpectedly, everything went terribly wrong. My wife appeared to be quite ill for a few weeks, and then left. Divorce followed faster than even Hollywood could muster, and in order to keep the house I sold the practice and sent the proceeds in their entirety to my 'ex' who was now in Canada with a man she had met on the Internet, remortgaged the house for an amount that took my breath away in order to pay her still more, and settled for a reduction in income of around a third, as I was now in the employment of two young dentists to whom I had sold the practice.

It was around Christmas time, and I found myself alone in the house. And then, wonderfully, the house was full of daughters, and son in law, and daughter's boyfriend, and we celebrated Christmas as best we could.

Friends would telephone and ask me out for a meal, which was so lovely of them, and others would get in touch and say, "Don't do anything stupid, will you? Not really stupid, I mean." But by the grace of God I am a survivor, and while those who knew me wondered just what would become of me after being financially plundered at such a critical time in life, there were some truly wonderful surprises just round the corner.

CHAPTER 10

Wonder Woman, Deserts, The Antarctic, and the Rabbit Family!

Life at the practice continued much as it had for some years; 'the usual drill' I used to call it. I liked my work and loved my patients – well, most of them. Hundreds of them had been with me for years, and I knew their families, knew where they holidayed, their hobbies, and so on and so forth. Every day was like a friends' reunion.

Suddenly finding myself alone the previous August had been quite a bombshell. I had been so worried about what was happening to my wife, as we had been very much in love for so many years. When she had left I did not give much thought to the financial aspects of the situation, as I was still so concerned for her. It had been my practice for decades to spend time daily reading the Bible and praying, and so I would now put aside a little while four or five times a day, read a psalm and pray. The fact that I tangibly received strength came home to me when two different and unrelated people used the same words in asking me, "How can you be so strong." Of course, they had not seen the tears and the heartbreak, but the Lord did make me strong. I did a course for people who had lost their partners through death, separation or divorce, and found that some of the people on it had waited two or three years before being able to face such sessions.

Some things I did were really sensible, such as spending more time with God. Some things were just props to help me through, such as the secondhand Jaguar XK8, a rather hairy sports car with drop dead good looks. Other things were sensible escapism, such as when I drove the Jaguar down to Switzerland to spend some days with a friend from our church, who had gone there to help build up a Swiss church, fallen in love and married.

The divorce had gone through, and I had to sit down and have a look at my finances, come to terms with a precarious situation, and make some plans for the future. Different people approach such matters in their own way, and some ways work and some do not. My method was to sit and make a list of things to do, and it was called something like 'Action!' It looked so spiritual, but item number one was 'Always put God first'. Impractical? Unrealistic? The way one sees it almost certainly depends on the way one sees God. And then there was advice for myself, such as, 'Dentistry is piece-work – don't talk so much', and 'Try and maintain a good relationship with the new practice owners – you need to keep working there', and so on.

I must confess that I rather like being married, though at this time I was not hunting for a wife. However, I did feel that I would like to marry again in a year or two, and drew up one or two things I would like to see in a new wife. One such item read, 'Born again Christian,' and another read 'Rich Widow!'

* * * * * * * * * *

One Sunday morning at our church, a lady went forward to the microphone and said she would like to speak about something she had learnt over the past few years. She started speaking, but as she did so a lady with a miniskirt pushed her away along the row, sat next to me, and whispered in my ear that I must be feeling rather rejected. "No," I whispered back, but she put her hand on my knee and said she had been through a difficult time herself. Now, you may feel that this lady had more in mind than helping me spiritually, but I knew her well and she in fact simply wanted to help me in that way.

Don't always judge by appearances! But I wanted to hear what the lady at the microphone was saying, and it was impossible with the whispering in my ear.

The lady speaking to the church was called Wendy. She had been a member even longer than me, and I had been there sixteen years. I did not know her at all, but I could remember her husband leaving her years before, and she had brought up two daughters single-handed. And I thought to myself, '*She's single!*'

That evening I telephoned her to ask what she had said at the microphone, and she told me that after her husband had left, she had looked for fulfilment in various ways, but had now found it by making her life around her God, her family, her home, her church and her work. My response to this was to ask her out to dinner, and a few days later I took her to a small restaurant by the riverside at a village called Horning. It was a pleasant evening, and she seemed a pleasant lady.

A few days later I felt rather despondent about my situation and decided I needed to get away for a few days. With a week-end approaching, France seemed to beckon, and a crazy thought entered my head – ask Wendy to come too.

"France for the day? What will we do in France?" asked Wendy over the telephone. "Have lunch," I replied, and she paused before saying, "OK, we'll do it."

"Bring an overnight bag," I said on the spur of the moment, "If lunch is no good, we'll need to stay and have another one!"

We drove down to Dover early on the Friday morning, caught the ferry to Calais and had one of the worst lunches ever (not by my arrangement!), and so we drove along the coast looking for a hotel with a sea view. At the town of Berck we found such a hotel, called La Littoral, and seemed to cause total confusion by asking for separate rooms. "Are you not together?" asked the proprietor, and I said we were. "Then, it is *one* – *une* - room," he replied, holding up one finger. "No," I said, "We want separate rooms. Two rooms – *deux*," holding up two fingers. "One each." "But you are together," he said, but after much shrugging of the shoulders, we were given two separate rooms.

We walked along the beach, and found we knew so much more about each other's families than we had realized. Wendy had worked as a nurse with Sheila at a hospital, and had known Dawn through the church. She had met my children in the church, and I had met her children in the church – and in the dental chair! We talked about our work, and our faith, and our interests – and we almost missed dinner. It was a great weekend, and Wendy later told me that in her heart she committed herself to me at that time. I am so glad she did not tell me then, as I was not ready for anything like that, and would have run!

I could make this a long story, but suffice to say that we had a romantic year. Wendy had brought up her daughters by working all hours as a nurse, and had been on just one holiday in eighteen years. So after France I took her whale-watching off Iceland, we spent time in Rome and Sorrento, and I introduced her to one of my most favourite places – Dovedale on the Derbyshire-Staffordshire border. I found that Wendy was not a rich widow, and I explained that my finances were rather precarious at that time, but we truly trusted God. Well, we married each other! Our first 'date' had been on the first of March 2002, and we married at our church on the first of March 2003. Wendy was a popular figure, admired for the way she had looked after her children so single-mindedly, and most people knew me as I had been there so many years, and preached and taught for much of that time. Around 350 people came to the wedding, and around 300 to the reception. We honeymooned on safari, which was one of Wendy's dreams, and I felt it was the best holiday I had ever had.

I had asked Wendy what her dreams were, and found that for financial reasons I was unable to make two of them come true at that time. But after a year or two I took her to see both the Great Wall of China and the Galapagos Islands to the west of the coast of South America. And she asked me *my* dreams, and I remembered that as a boy I had always wanted to go to the Antarctic. So we flew to Argentina and sailed, first to the Falklands and South Georgia, and then on to the Antarctic, where we walked on the Peninsula and sailed through to the Weddell Sea until there was pack ice. Returning by Cape Horn we encountered a force 12 gale that caused considerable damage to the ship internally and put a few people in hospital. Wendy did not call these times holidays, but *adventures*, and we have adopted that term ever since.

South America became one of 'our places', though we often found ourselves there with two other couples we had first met in the Galapagos Islands, and in addition to scrambling up mountains, usually the Andes, and trekking through parts of Patagonia, we explored a few deserts, flying over the Nazca Lines in the Nazca desert in Peru, and spending some time in the Atacama desert, admiring its rugged arid sculpted profile, salt flats, and the Valley of the Moon.

* * * * * * * * * *

"You've got a hairy nose," said a small child looking up from the chair. Children can be embarrassingly uninhibited at times, and I saw the mother cringe as the child spoke. But I was used to this, and simply responded, "Yes, very hairy."

I reflected on some of the other incidents involving children over the years. Some patients wrote me really nice letters to say how much they had appreciated their treatment at the practice, and others sent me cards. I kept all these in albums in case I ever received a complaining letter and needed to boost my self-confidence. At Christmas bottles of various descriptions were delivered to reception, and many of those containing spirits are still enjoyed by guests and visitors to our home, as I find them a little too strong for me. And one letter arrived from a lad of around twelve years, who had attended for the extraction of four teeth prior to orthodontic work. The letter simply read –

"*Dear Uncle Barrie, You are a good tooth puller outer. Love from Jordan*"

On another occasion a lady had attended to have a tooth prepared for a crown, and brought her small daughter Emily with her, who stood in the corner of the surgery holding her dolly and looking through a Ladybird book. She returned two weeks later to have the crown fitted, and it was the technician's practice to send the porcelain crown in a small glass container, having cotton wool at the bottom, the crown laying on it, with more cotton wool on top. Emily and dolly just stood and watched from the corner again. I removed the lid of the container, and said, "Your tooth should be ready for you today." I removed the cotton wool from the top part of the container, but could not see the crown, and so removed the rest of the cotton wool. Still no crown. "It must be hiding in the cotton wool," I said to the mother, and continued to feel through the cotton wool that was now on the worktop. And then I realized – the technician, for the first time ever, had forgotten to place the crown in the container.

I looked at the patient, and said, "I'm terribly sorry. Your tooth is not in the container."

Before I could proceed to explain what I thought had happened, a little lisping voice piped up from the corner of the surgery.

"I ecthpect the toof fairy has taken it Mr. Lawrence!"

That was one of the sweetest moments of my career, and said in such innocence. But one or two other stories involving children were not so lovely. A lad of around twelve was brought to the practice by his big brother of about sixteen, and he accompanied him into my upstairs surgery.

"What can I do for you," I asked, and he replied, "I'm scared."

"There's nothing to worry about seeing me," I said, trying to reassure the boy, but he simply jumped out of the chair, opened the surgery door and ran. He sounded like thunder racing down the stairs.

"I'll get 'im," shouted the brother, and there was a sound of even louder thunder as he tumbled down the stairs and gave chase. I assumed that we would not see either of them again for a month or two, and said to the nurse, "Time for a coffee, I think."

Barely three minutes into our coffee there was a sound of groaning and pleading from the staircase, and we walked through to the waiting room to find the younger lad with a cut on his face, and possible bruising, being dragged towards the surgery door by his older brother.

"Got 'im," he announced triumphantly. "Got 'im with a rugger tackle outside the fruit shop on the corner. Here 'e is mate." But dental treatment seemed totally inappropriate by now, and we cleaned up the younger boy and put a dressing on his face, and gave the older boy a severe lecture on how to behave towards younger family members.

On another occasion, I might have been the one receiving the lecture. It had been the early days at the Norwich practice, and the surgery was on the ground floor at the front of the building, looking out onto the road. The lower half of the window had frosted glass so that people could not see in. However, some of the local youngsters would creep up to the window, and climb onto the window sill so that they could stare in through the unfrosted top half of the window. And then they would shout at me, and I would swing round to see them laughing. They would jump down and scamper off along the road.

One afternoon after school time, I was aware of a shadow behind the frosted glass of the lower part of the window, and as there was not a patient in the surgery, decided to have a little fun. Grasping a pair of extraction forceps, I moved back and hid to one side of the window. I was soon aware of small faces peering in through the top half of the window, and suddenly leapt out from the side of the window, waving my forceps a few inches in front of their faces, shouting "Gonna get you!"

There were loud shrieks as small boys fell off the window sill and ran for their lives. Not surprisingly, that was the last time they troubled me in that way at the surgery, but I do wonder if they went through life telling people, "You'll never guess why I'm afraid of the dentist......"

* * * * * * * * * *

Wendy had lived in a small two-bedroomed cottage that had originally been built for workers at the local water-mill. It was beautiful, but small. I would have liked us to retain it as a holiday cottage, or to let out. Not only was it her family home of many years, but also just five minutes' walk from the local Indian restaurant! Were we to sell our respective homes and buy somewhere new, or move into Wendy's home or mine? With six daughters, Wendy's home would have limitations for our enlarged family, and yet mine had associations with the past. However, I had six bedrooms, and a multitude of downstairs rooms, as I had twice extended the property since acquiring it as a two-bedroomed cottage.

Our decision was to sell Wendy's cottage and to move into mine, and for Wendy to redecorate throughout in order to stamp her personality and taste onto our new home. We also changed some of the furniture, and Wendy had a new bathroom and kitchen designed and installed.

We have six daughters and four sons-in-law. One daughter is a widow, and one has a long-term partner. At the time of writing we have 17 grandchildren. To make matters a little bit more complicated, our six daughters live in five different countries, though two live in England. Once recently, we have had all daughters and grandchildren, and some sons-in-law staying here, which has meant sleeping twenty-three and feeding twenty seven. Wendy positively enthuses over these times, and is known to many of our friends as 'Wonder Woman', or 'WWW' which stands for Wonder Woman Wendy! There seem to be so many of us; it reminds me of 'The Rabbit Family' from a childhood storybook.

The plan had once been that my previous wife and I would retire, sell the practice and pay off the mortgage. Also, our home needed a new roof. Now everything had changed. Since our marriage, Wendy had experienced rapid promotion in the residential home where she had worked as a nurse, and found herself as manager. The question for us was, when should we retire? I was reluctant – I liked my work and I loved my patients, so how would I cope emotionally without that aspect of my life? My financial position had changed dramatically, as not only had my practice gone and the mortgage doubled, but also some of my pensions had been sent to Canada as part of the settlement. But Wendy and I have a Father in heaven who cares for His children on earth, and we felt that there were many things for us to be busy with that only retirement would really permit. I arranged a date for this with the young couple who had bought my practice, and though Wendy decided to retire at the same time, the home she managed was suddenly closed because of a change in business emphasis by the company owning it. So by March 2007 we found ourselves with so much more time on our hands.

Have you heard retired people say, "I'm so busy now that I don't know how I found time to work?" We had heard that so many times, but found in our own experience that it is quite true.

Leaving our church after twenty-five years of membership because of a vivid dream we believed was from the Lord, does seem so 'whacky' – but at the time of writing we have had a church meeting in our home for over two years. Most of us who meet together have been damaged by life in one way or another, but many of us have, by the grace of God, come through and recovered. We seek to help and encourage one another as we meet with the living God who can really restore those who are broken. At the time of writing, around 130 people have been through our sitting room, though only a minority has stayed, and we are soon moving out into a small hall.

Attending a few dinners of the local Full Gospel Business-men's Fellowship was intended to give us occasional experience of wider fellowship with Christians of various denominations and none – but I quickly found myself central to that work, and in addition to presiding over monthly dinners of up to a hundred people, Wonder Woman gives a monthly supper at our home attended by up to thirty five people (attracted partly, I feel sure, by the choice of four different hot main courses). We also travel to different parts of the country speaking at evangelistic meetings and dinners. Getting to know the village has involved an open breakfast invitation to local people, and over fifty attended. And then after three weeks of spare-time scribbling in 2012, my first book was 'born', and the very first publishers I approached offered me a contract. This led to further activity, particularly evangelistic speaking engagements and book signings. I also continue to do after-dinner speaking, and similar engagements when invited, simply to entertain.

As a lad I had decided that my working life would be involved with holey teeth. I would never have guessed where that road would lead, with the adventure of training as a dentist at the London Hospital and of the life-changing experience of coming to Christ as my Saviour and Lord. I had assumed that I would have a surgery in a High Street somewhere, but to end up having seven surgeries and a bookshop was beyond my imagination. I had also assumed that I would marry, settle down, have two children and one day retire and sit by the fire doting on grandchildren who would live a short drive away. When we are young there are things in life, which 'only happen to other people,' but the harsh reality of life is that they can happen to me, happen to us, and happen to you, the reader. The God I read about in the pages of the Bible is the One who has seen me through the valleys and mountaintops of life as a dentist, bookseller, husband, father and grandfather; the One Who has made all of life 'holy', including my patients' teeth (if you will excuse the pun). I commend Him to every one of you, my readers.

Appendix 1

Some Dental Jokes

There seems to be something funny about false teeth, and people even give suppressed giggles when I enthuse over the blood and gore of removing obstinate wisdom teeth. Others just cringe or leave the room, and so I have learnt to be sensitive and diplomatic (to some extent) over the years.

From my early days as a dental student I started collecting dental cartoons from newspapers and magazines, as the subject has obviously appealed to others too. I have also kept in mind various dental jokes that I have heard during my years in the profession, and still occasionally hear one that is new to me. And I have made up a few of my own. Many of my patients seemed to appreciate hearing them, or were polite, or scared stiff of offending me by not laughing. Below I have written a few of them, most of which are as old as the hills, some as old as Tommy Cooper would have been, and some from the author himself!

* * *

Question: What do you call a man who has had a tooth prepared for a crown?
Answer: Spike!

* * *

Question: What do you call a woman with a tooth prepared for a crown?
Answer: Peggy!

* * *

Question: What do you call a lady who has her front tooth missing?
Answer: Bridget!

* * *

Question: Why does a man with just his front teeth left, never feel the cold?
Answer: Because he's got central 'eating!

* * *

Question: What award does the 'Dentist of the Year' get?
Answer: A little plaque!

* * *

Question: What did the dentist say to the golfer?
Answer: You have a hole in one!

* * *

Question: Why did the dentist seem sad?
Answer: Because he looked down in the mouth!

* * *

Question: Has your tooth stopped hurting yet?
Answer: I don't know. The dentist kept it!

* * *

Question: What time is your appointment with the dentist?
Answer: Tooth Hurty!

* * *

Patient to dentist – "Hey dentist, your last chair used to go up and down. This one goes backwards and forwards."
Dentist to patient – "Get out of my filing cabinet!"

* * *

Dentist to patient – "Now stick your tongue out, and without smiling say Aaaaahhhhhhhhh!"
Patient to dentist – "What does that tell you then, dentist?"
Dentist to patient – "It tells me nothing, but my cat died this morning."

* * *

A man is invited to be guest speaker at a rather formal dinner, and arrives at the venue, makes conversation with those present, and sits down to enjoy the meal. As he starts to eat he realizes that he has left his false teeth at home, and that he will lisp and be unable to smile during his speech. Turning to the man on his left, he says, "I've left my teef at home."
The man on his left says, "Oh dear, what are you going to do?"
He turns to the man on his right, and says, "I've left my teef at home."
The man on his right says, "Never mind. I can help you," and fumbling in his left-hand jacket pocket, produces a set of false teeth, saying 'Try these."
They feel really clumsy and hurt, so he says, "They're no good. They don't fit and they hurt me."
"No problem," says the man on his right, and fumbling through the same pocket, brings out another set of false teeth, "Try these," he says.
"Ouch – they hurt too. They dig in," says the guest speaker, and removes them.
"No problem at all," says the other man, and puts his hand in his left-hand trouser pocket. "Try these."
This time they rattle all round the inside of his mouth, and he spits them out into his hand, explaining that these too do not fit.

"No problem old chap," says his companion, and putting his hand in his right-hand trouser pocket, says "Try these."

"What are you?" enquires the guest speaker. "Are you a dentist?"

"No," replied the man on his right, "I'm an undertaker!"

* * *

A man walks into a dental surgery, and says to the dentist, "Hello. How are you today?"

The dentist looks blank, shrugs his shoulders and says nothing.

"I just wanted to know how you are," said the patient. "Been anywhere interesting this year? Any holidays?"

Again the dentist looks blank, shrugs his shoulders and says nothing.

The patient gives a sigh of resignation, climbs into the chair, and leaning his head back, opens his mouth. The dentist duly starts looking round the teeth with his mirror and probe well into the orifice. However, the patient decides to have one last try at greeting the dentist and enquiring as to his health and any recent excursions, but manages to simply make a succession of incoherent sounds.

"Eeerrrrr splu'er, ch'ke, uuummmmmm, owwww splutter, are, cough, errrrr........." he emits.

These sounds are immediately recognized by the dentist, who smiles broadly and says, "I'm fine thanks. Really well. Yes, we had a little cruise round the Caribbean and a week or two in the sun in Spain. How about you?" and continues, obliviously, to check round the teeth.

* * *

Patient: How much do you charge to extract a wisdom tooth?
Dentist: It will be in the region of £250.
Patient: That's ridiculous! Isn't there something cheaper?
Dentist: I could extract it for £150 if I don't use anaesthetic.
Patient: No way. That's still way too much.

Dentist: OK. If I just rip it out with pliers, the price will be £50.
Patient: That's more like it. Book my husband in for next Monday.

* * *

A man goes to the dentist for a check-up. The dentist looks in his mouth, and says –
"There's a tremendous cavity in this tooth. There's a tremendous cavity in this tooth."
"OK," said the patient, "You don't have to repeat it."
"I didn't," said the dentist. "That was the echo!"

* * *

A new dentist in town quickly gained a reputation for being absolutely painless. A young lad made an appointment and went to see the dentist. When he came out, he said, "He's not painless at all. I bit his finger hard and he yelled like anyone else!"

* * *

And remember – you don't have to brush all of your teeth; just the ones you want to keep!

* * *

Did you hear about the chiropodist who married a dentist? They opened a foot and mouth clinic!

Appendix 2

The Key

It was sometime during my first term at the London, at a social event, that a medical student said to me in conversation, "Jesus Christ has changed my life." I was not sure how to respond, but I know what I thought - "You poor boy. You want to be a *doctor*? Man, you need to *see* a doctor!"

That incident left me wondering why an intelligent, really decent person would say something like that. No one I had met in churches had ever said anything like that, though my mother had warned me about 'Holy Joes'! And then I met Sheila, and a little later it seemed that intelligent decent people with real faith and experience of God were everywhere. Why did they say this? I was an atheist, and believed there was no God or gods. Could I possibly be wrong? Only a fool would ignore or dismiss such an issue, and you have read 'what happened next' in this book.

I could use a lot of religious jargon to try and explain just how different life is after being 'born again' - which itself could be called religious jargon. Suffice to say that I have felt so *fulfilled* - a sort of job satisfaction in living. I used to be something of a complainer; my glass was half empty, and life was not what I kept hoping it would be. Suddenly, my glass was at worst half-full, and so often full to overflowing.

I have known heartbreak, rejection, disappointment, and disillusionment (not least with myself); my finances have been precarious at times; occasionally I have been almost overwhelmed with grief. And yet, I trust that something of my 'new life', which makes me (in Bible language) 'more than a conqueror' and 'an overcomer', comes through in my writing. Truly, the God I read about in the Bible is alive, real, powerful, compassionate, and he speaks to us. And there is so much more. I have been miraculously healed and seen miracles in other people's lives too. On many occasions I have had instant and amazing answers to prayer. Not all the time - but often.

In this book I have written a short autobiography for you, and I trust you have enjoyed it. Yes - *enjoyed*. But don't miss the most important and vital part, which is integral to my story - that the quality of life I enjoy in this world of difficulty, trial and heartbreak, flows from a real relationship with the one true God. And quite simply, what he's done for me he can do for anyone - maybe you? In my book *There Must be More to Life Than This!*, I have written more fully of my experience of the God of the Bible, and it includes a reader-friendly guide on how anyone can live such an enriched and fulfilling life.

I wish you much joy and big blessings!

VIPs

"Write a book, Barrie!" said Toby Lewis, probably our favourite patient, exuding his inimitable charm and grace. "Write a book!" said countless members of dinner clubs, luncheon clubs, associations, fellowships, Women's' Institutes, as well as those attending dinners of a major political party where I had spoken a time or three to entertain them. I thank them all for their encouragement, and especially Toby.

"Not *another* book!" said one or two of my friends. I think they were encouraging me, and if so, I thank them too.

It is proper and appropriate, as well as courteous, to thank people who have been helpful and kind, or who have simply helped one along in life, and especially so with an autobiography. But where does one draw the line without omitting a deserving case? So, it's family and people mentioned in the text, and people who have helped directly with production of the book - and a few others.

If it had not been for my parents, there would be no Barrie and no story. Thank you, mother and father, for bringing me into this world, tolerating frogs and mice in our home, coaching me academically for the eleven-plus exam, and encouraging me to pursue a career in dentistry. And my sister was quite tolerant too - thank you Julia.

Blue Year - you were, and continue to be - GREAT! I loved your company, humour, support, encouragement, and again - toleration. I continue to appreciate you deeply, as none of us have changed a scrap since we first met. To those of you I have paraded across some of these pages, please forgive me. To those of you I have omitted, please forgive me.

To my many thousands of patients through several decades, I am truly grateful to you and love you. From sitting members of the upper house and leaders of British industry, to those like myself of humbler station in this world, you have enriched my life with personality, conversation, humour and concern. "Have you heard the one about....." was always appreciated, and those who said "Come out for a drink sometime," at times of grief were simply friends *disguised* as patients. Like Blue Year, I have preserved your anonymity (thinly in the case of Blue Year) by changing your names. Again, forgive me if you would have preferred stardom, but discretion is the better part of valour, so I've been told.

Political correctness has not been a great forté of mine, and I want to thank my proofreaders for saving me from the gallows, in addition to correcting grammar and spelling, and helping iron out hesitation, deviation and repetition. Cameron Duffy, has again excelled at spotting Grandad's errors, and I'm grateful for the time given by such a busy and intelligent young man. Sharon Dancu, who I have known as a FaceBook friend for some months, has given hours and hours to combing through the manuscript, and bringing to my attention both errors, and ideas with regard to enhancing the nature of the presentation. Sharon is now a professional proofreader, and can be contacted at sdanc@uwclub.net. Finally, Stephen Scott-Fawcett made innumerable suggestions with regard to grammar and to generally 'embellishing the literary style'. I am greatly indebted to Steve for this, and for the Foreword – but more on that below.

Derek Blois has been a friend for nearly thirty years now, and has been there with encouragement and support at critical times in my life. But Derek is also an artist, and advised me with regard to my previous book. "Change the title," he said. "I wouldn't buy it with *that* title!" We used his new title, and people have loved it. And again Derek has excelled with a magnificent cover for this book. Derek, Maestro, you are amazing, and I am truly grateful to you. You can view some of his magnificent paintings at http://www.picturecraftgallery.co.uk/derek-blois/

The Foreword. Stephen Scott-Fawcett has been a friend and an inspiration for a long time. We are all unique, but Steve is more unique than most! Walking to both poles, climbing Everest and other 'Himalayan hills' (Steve's modest description of huge mountains), trekking his beloved Nepal sometimes with his gentle-hearted and beautiful wife Laxmi, and training native pastors in evangelism, healing and deliverance makes my life seem very safe and simple. I am indebted to Steve for his kindness in writing a foreword to this book, and emailing it from Pokhara in Nepal. When it arrived, I was rather busy, but having read the first few words, felt compelled to sit down and read it aloud to Wendy. We hooted with laughter several times, but more importantly were so impressed with the erudite and scholarly quality of the writing. Steve edits the James Caird Society *Journal*, and has recently published *The Shackleton Centenary Book (2014)*. You can read more on this at www.jamescairdsociety.com/ journal

My four daughters have encouraged me in all things good, and most things mischievous (on whom did we drop sugar lumps from our hotel window in St. Helier? Ah Yes, 'twas the headwaiter and anyone else passing by) and I adore each of you and your wonderful families. As I have said, Wendy and I have six daughters living in five different countries, and girls - you are fantastic. That is why we keep visiting you, but I want to say 'Thank you' to Sarah, Rachel, Naomi, Deborah, Fiona and Heather - you are simply *kind* to me, and you said *kind* and *lovely* things about my last book. Don't stop now!

May I mention my first wife Sheila? You helped lead me to faith in Christ, and we enjoyed romance and marriage. You gave me four beautiful daughters and we enjoyed family together. Thank you for everything, and I wish you joy.

Dawn - we enjoyed romance, dentistry, bookshop, holidays and our dear little cottage, which grew and grew. Thank you for everything, and I wish you joy.

Don Double has been a 'spiritual father' to me for many years, and I am grateful to him and his late wife Heather for their love and care. Wonderful people!

Wendy is known to some of my friends as 'WWW', which stands for 'Wonder Woman Wendy', so I am told. Life is a journey, and I have experienced the valleys and the mountain peaks, the grief and the exhilaration. I was emerging from 'Valley of Grief Number 2' when you came on the scene, and you were a gift from God. The Lord has always been good to me, but especially in bringing you into my life. Because of you, my latter years are full of contentment and deep joy, in finding romance, companionship and a true partner in everything that matters. Praying together and cuddling together, walking, cooking, serving in the church, entertaining multitudes, and enjoying the countless sensible, stupid, intelligent and downright ridiculous things that make our lives so full, is a joy I never expected and do not deserve. You are one big 'WOW' (as well as 'WWW') and I thank you from the bottom of my heart. Understatement.

When I came to faith in Christ, I was changed. HE changed me. He fulfilled me, and continues to do so. To quote a certain Terry Eckersley, he turned my mess into a message, and my tests into testimonies. I thank and praise the Lord Jesus for giving me Life with a capital 'L', and if you don't understand this, please read *There Must be More to Life Than This!* or drop me an email.

To you, the reader, thank you for coming thus far. If you have enjoyed it, tell your friends. And if you have not - hush! But I truly hope that you have.

THERE MUST BE MORE TO LIFE THAN THIS!
How to know the God of the Bible in Everyday Life

by Barrie Lawrence

Published by New Wine Press

Barrie writes in his own distinctive style of incidents in his life that can only be described as amazing coincidences – or acts of God!

Three radiographers had declared that the man's arm was broken and it was encased in plaster. Of course it was! So how was he out of plaster and using it normally less than a week later? On another occasion Barrie sent a paperback book to a patient, as he thought it would be helpful. The patient's wife took it from the postman, panicked, and called the emergency services to say a bomb had just been delivered. Why? And there was the boy in Mexico whose arm had been fixed with plates and screws when it had been fractured a year earlier. Barrie and Wendy were called to the school and asked to perform a miracle, to make the arm work normally again – and the whole class waited to see the wonder! Read of the amazing outcome, but be prepared to be challenged in your thinking.

Not without humour, Barrie writes of the ways *he* has been challenged on various occasions in his life, of his successes and his failures. It's OK to laugh at him at times, because he does so himself, but you may also want to weep with him as he opens his heart about coping with difficulties and heartbreaks. Above all, it is an inspiring book that seeks to lift the reader onto a higher plane in life.

The first half of the book, part one, comprises fifteen short chapters of true stories from Barrie's own life, while part two has a clear message – it's happened to me and it can happen to you. In fact, part two is a reader-friendly guide to help anyone to come to know the God who we read about in the Bible.

If there are times when you think to yourself "There must be more to life than this," then this book is a *must-read* for you!

Available from www.amazon.co.uk and all good bookshops.